ABC OF WOUND HEALING

Edited by

JOSEPH E GREY
Consultant physician, University Hospital of Wales, Cardiff and Vale NHS Trust, and honorary consultant in wound healing, Wound Healing Research Unit, Cardiff University

and

KEITH G HARDING
Head of the Wound Healing Research Unit, Cardiff University, and professor and honorary consultant in rehabilitation medicine (wound healing), Cardiff and Vale NHS Trust and Gwent NHS Trust

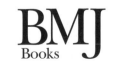

BMJ
Books

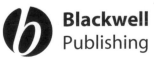

Blackwell
Publishing

© 2006 by Blackwell Publishing Ltd
BMJ Books is an imprint of the BMJ Publishing Group Limited, used under licence

Blackwell Publishing, Inc., 350 Main Street, Malden, Massachusetts 02148-5020, USA
Blackwell Publishing Ltd, 9600 Garsington Road, Oxford OX4 2DQ, UK
Blackwell Publishing Asia Pty Ltd, 550 Swanston Street, Carlton, Victoria 3053, Australia

First published 2006

3   2007

Library of Congress Cataloging-in-Publication Data
ABC of wound healing / edited by Joseph E. Grey, Keith G. Harding.
        p. : cm.
    "BMJ Books."
    Includes bibliographical references and index.
    ISBN-13: 978-0-7279-1695-2 (alk.paper)
    ISBN-10: 0-7279-1695-5 (alk.paper)
    1. Wound healing—Handbooks, manuals, etc. 2. Wounds and injuries—Treatment—
Handbooks, manuals, etc. I. Grey, Joseph E. II. Harding, K. G. (Keith G.)
    [DNLM: 1. Wounds and Injuries—therapy—Handbooks. 2. Ulcer—therapy—
Handbooks. 3. Wound Healing—physiology—Handbooks. 4. Wounds and Injuries—
diagnosis—Handbooks. WO 39 A134 2006]
    RD94.A23 2006
    617.1—dc22

                                                                    2006013655

ISBN-13: 978 0 7279 1695 2

A catalogue record for this title is available from the British Library

The cover shows a scanning electron micrograph of a healing wound on the skin, five
days after injury. With permission from Eye of Science/Science Photo Library

Set by BMJ Electronic Production
Printed and bound in Spain by GraphyCems

Commissioning Editor: Eleanor Lines
Editorial Assistant: Victoria Pittman
Senior Technical Editor: Julia Thompson
Development Editors: Sally Carter/Nick Morgan
Production Controller: Debbie Wyer

For further information on Blackwell Publishing, visit our website:
http://www.blackwellpublishing.com

The publisher's policy is to use permanent paper from mills that operate a sustainable forestry policy,
and which has been manufactured from pulp processed using acid-free and elementary chlorine-free
practices. Furthermore, the publisher ensures that the text paper and cover board used have met
acceptable environmental accreditation standards.

Contents

Contributors   iv

Preface   v

1   **Wound assessment**   1
Joseph E Grey, Stuart Enoch, Keith G Harding

2   **Venous and arterial leg ulcers**   5
Joseph E Grey, Stuart Enoch, Keith G Harding

3   **Diabetic foot ulcers**   9
Michael E Edmonds, A V M Foster

4   **Pressure ulcers**   13
Joseph E Grey, Stuart Enoch, Keith G Harding

5   **Traumatic and surgical wounds**   17
David J Leaper, Keith G Harding

6   **Uncommon causes of ulceration**   21
Girish K Patel, Joseph E Grey, Keith G Harding

7   **Burns**   24
Alex Benson, William A Dickson, Dean E Boyce

8   **Reconstructive surgery**   28
Dean E Boyce, Kayvan Shokrollahi

9   **Wound dressings**   31
Vanessa Jones, Joseph E Grey, Keith G Harding

10   **Infections**   35
Brendan Healy, Andrew Freedman

11   **Non-surgical and drug treatments**   39
Stuart Enoch, Joseph E Grey, Keith G Harding

12   **Recent advances and emerging treatments**   43
Stuart Enoch, Joseph E Grey, Keith G Harding

Index   47

Contributors

Alex Benson
Specialist registrar in plastic surgery, Mersey Regional Plastic Surgery Unit, Whiston Hospital, Liverpool

Dean E Boyce
Consultant hand and plastic surgeon, Welsh Centre for Burns and Plastic Surgery, Morriston Hospital, Swansea

William A Dickson
Consultant burns and plastic surgeon, Welsh Centre for Burns and Plastic Surgery, Morriston Hospital, Swansea

Michael E Edmonds
Consultant physician, Diabetic Foot Clinic, King's College Hospital, London

Stuart Enoch
Research Fellow of the Royal College of Surgeons of England, Wound Healing Research Unit, Cardiff University, Cardiff

A V M Foster
Chief podiatrist, Diabetic Foot Clinic, King's College Hospital, London

Andrew Freedman
Honorary consultant in infectious diseases, University Hospital of Wales, Cardiff

Joseph E Grey
Consultant physician, University Hospital of Wales, Cardiff and Vale NHS Trust, and honorary consultant in wound healing, Wound Healing Research Unit, Cardiff University, Cardiff

Keith G Harding
Head of the Wound Healing Research Unit, Cardiff University, and professor and honorary consultant in rehabilitation medicine (wound healing), Cardiff and Vale NHS Trust and Gwent NHS Trust

Brendan Healy
Specialist registrar in infectious diseases and microbiology, University Hospital of Wales, Cardiff

Vanessa Jones
Senior lecturer, Wound Healing Research Unit, Cardiff University, Cardiff

David J Leaper
Visiting professor of surgery, Wound Healing Research Unit, Cardiff University, Cardiff

Girish K Patel
Research fellow in wound healing and honorary clinical tutor in dermatology, Cardiff University and Cardiff and Vale NHS Trust, Cardiff

Kayvan Shokrollahi
Specialist registrar in plastic surgery, Welsh Centre for Burns and Plastic Surgery, Morriston Hospital, Swansea

Preface

Wounds have existed since the beginning of time. Increasingly bloody conflicts have led to improved management of traumatic wounds and the development of new surgical approaches and disciplines such as plastic surgery. However, many patients with wounds experience difficulties in accessing clinicians with an interest and expertise in this common and costly aspect of clinical practice.

Despite advances in surgical techniques and the use of antibiotic prophylaxis, approximately 10% of patients who undergo 'clean' operations develop surgical site infections. Up to 15% of health service costs are devoted to the treatment of diabetes: the most expensive component is the management of diabetic foot disease, the most likely reason for such patients to be admitted to hospital. Around 4% of NHS costs are spent on the prevention and treatment of pressure ulcers. Increasing litigation activity associated with this wound type compounds the financial burden.

Wounds are diverse in nature and are likely to require a number of interventions to ensure optimal care. Perhaps the major reason for a lack of progress in this subject, until recently, is the lack of multi-professional teams working in an interdisciplinary way to ensure all relevant skills and expertise are available to the individual with a wound.

The *ABC of Wound Healing* series attempts to provide clinicians, from all professional backgrounds, with an insight into a range of issues associated with wounds. The first chapter deals with wound assessment, a basic component of care since patients are unlikely to receive appropriate treatment and achieve a reasonable outcome if both patient and the wound are not assessed in an appropriate manner.

Subsequent chapters deal with specific wound types, both chronic and acute in nature, whilst the final part provides information regarding treatment ranging from dressings, devices, drugs, surgery, physical, chemical and on to biological and emerging therapies for patients with wounds.

Many of the authors of the chapters in this series are based in Wales. This is not because there is a monopoly of expertise in this area in the principality but rather is a reflection of the work of a large number of individuals who have either worked in or have had links with the Wound Healing Research Unit in Cardiff University. This group is the product of the vision of Professor Les Hughes, now retired as Professor of Surgery in Cardiff, and has led to the creation of a large academically based and clinically focused group that has worked in a number of areas of wound healing. This group is a key component of the Cardiff Institute of Tissue Engineering and Repair (CITER), an even larger and more broadly based interdisciplinary research institute that has an interest in tissue repair in a variety of organs in the body. More recently, an All Wales Network in Burns and Tissue Repair (Ffenics) has been set up.

The subjects contained within the book are written by people who have an interest and expertise in their areas. They are comprehensive summaries of many years experience and we would like to thank all of the authors and their colleagues for providing educational material of such quality. We would particularly like to express our thanks to Dr Stuart Enoch for his enthusiastic support, for helping to maintain our focus and for his unstinting encouragement in the pursuit of the project.

We recognise that much more work is needed to ensure patients with wounds receive optimal care. We believe this book provides the basic information necessary to increase the knowledge base for clinicians. However, we also need to develop skills and modify existing attitudes in the management of patients with wounds if we are to complete the educational journey that is required.

Keith G Harding
Joseph F Grey

1 Wound assessment

Joseph E Grey, Stuart Enoch, Keith G Harding

Most wounds, of whatever aetiology, heal without difficulty. Some wounds, however, are subject to factors that impede healing, although these do not prevent healing if the wounds are managed appropriately. A minority of wounds will become chronic and non-healing. In these cases the ultimate goal is to control the symptoms and prevent complications, rather than healing the wound.

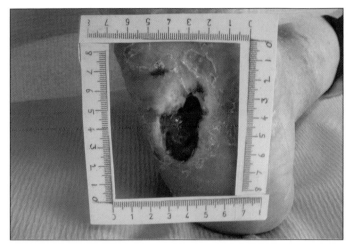

Wounds are not just skin deep, and accurate assessment is an essential part of treatment

Causes of ulceration

- Vascular (venous, arterial, lymphatic, vasculitis)
- Neuropathic (for example, diabetes, spina bifida, leprosy)
- Metabolic (for example, diabetes, gout)
- Connective tissue disease (for example, rheumatoid arthritis, scleroderma, systemic lupus erythematosus)
- Pyoderma gangrenosum (often reflection of systemic disorder)
- Haematological disease (red blood cell disorders (for example, sickle cell disease); white blood cell disorders (for example, leukaemia); platelet disorders (for example, thrombocytosis))
- Dysproteinaemias (for example, cryoglobulinaemia, amyloidosis)
- Immunodeficiency (for example, HIV, immunosuppressive therapy)
- Neoplastic (for example, basal cell carcinoma, squamous cell carcinoma, metastatic disease)
- Infectious (bacterial, fungal, viral)
- Panniculitis (for example, necrobiosis lipoidica)
- Traumatic (for example, pressure ulcer, radiation damage)
- Iatrogenic (for example, drugs)
- Factitious (self harm, "dermatitis artefacta")
- Others (for example, sarcoidosis)

It is important that the normal processes of developing a diagnostic hypothesis are followed before trying to treat the wound. A detailed clinical history should include information on the duration of ulcer, previous ulceration, history of trauma, family history of ulceration, ulcer characteristics (site, pain, odour, and exudate or discharge), limb temperature, underlying medical conditions (for example, diabetes mellitus, peripheral vascular disease, ischaemic heart disease, cerebrovascular accident, neuropathy, connective tissue diseases (such as rheumatoid arthritis), varicose veins, deep venous thrombosis), previous venous or arterial surgery, smoking, medications, and allergies to drugs and dressings. Appropriate investigations should be carried out.

Local and systemic factors that impede wound healing

Local factors	Systemic factors
- Inadequate blood supply	- Advancing age and general immobility
- Increased skin tension	- Obesity
- Poor surgical apposition	- Smoking
- Wound dehiscence	- Malnutrition
- Poor venous drainage	- Deficiency of vitamins and trace elements
- Presence of foreign body and foreign body reactions	- Systemic malignancy and terminal illness
	- Shock of any cause
	- Chemotherapy and radiotherapy
- Continued presence of micro-organisms	- Immunosuppressant drugs, corticosteroids, anticoagulants
- Infection	- Inherited neutrophil disorders, such as leucocyte adhesion deficiency
- Excess local mobility, such as over a joint	- Impaired macrophage activity (malacoplakia)

Some complications of chronic wounds

- Sinus formation
- Fistula
- Unrecognised malignancy
- Malignant transformation in the ulcer bed (Marjolin's ulcer)
- Osteomyelitis
- Contractures and deformity in surrounding joints
- Systemic amyloidosis
- Heterotopic calcification
- Colonisation by multiple drug resistant pathogens, leading to antibiotic resistance
- Anaemia
- Septicaemia

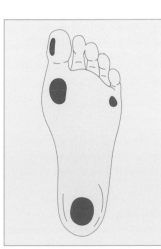

Areas of abnormal pressure distribution in the diabetic foot. Plantar ulcers are most commonly seen under the hallux, on the first and fifth metatarsal heads, and under the heel

Assessing wounds

Size of wound

The size of the wound should be assessed at first presentation and regularly thereafter. The outline of the wound margin should be traced on to transparent acetate sheets and the surface area estimated: in wounds that are approximately circular, multiply the longest diameter in one plane by the longest diameter in the plane at right angles; in irregularly shaped wounds, add up the number of squares contained within the margin of the outline of the wound from an acetate grid tracing. These methods are the simplest, but it should be recognised that they are not precise. However, they do provide a means by which progress over time to wound closure can be identified. Patient positioning, body curvature, or tapering of the limbs will affect the accuracy of these techniques.

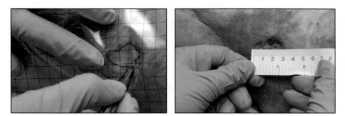

Tracing a wound for measurement and measuring a wound

Edge of wound

Although not diagnostic, examination of the edge of the wound may help to identify its aetiology in the context of the history of the wound. For example, venous leg ulcers generally have gently sloping edges, arterial ulcers often appear well demarcated and "punched out," and rolled or everted edges should raise the suspicion of malignancy. A biopsy should be taken of any suspicious wound.

Wound edge characteristics

Edges	Type of ulcer
Sloping	Venous ulcer
Punched out	Arterial or vasculitic ulcer
Rolled	Basal cell carcinoma
Everted	Squamous cell carcinoma
Undermining	Tuberculosis, syphilis
Purple	Vasculitic (such as pyoderma gangrenosum)

Site of wound

The site of the wound may aid diagnosis; diabetic foot ulcers often arise in areas of abnormal pressure distribution arising from disordered foot architecture. Venous ulceration occurs mostly in the gaiter area of the leg (see next article in this series). Non-healing ulcers, sometimes in unusual sites, should prompt consideration of malignancy.

Wound bed

Healthy granulation tissue is pink in colour and is an indicator of healing. Unhealthy granulation is dark red in colour, often bleeds on contact, and may indicate the presence of wound infection. Such wounds should be cultured and treated in the light of microbiological results. Excess granulation or overgranulation may also be associated with infection or non-healing wounds. These often respond to simple cautery with silver nitrate or with topically applied steroid preparations. Chronic wounds may be covered by white or yellow shiny

Laboratory investigations before treating a wound

Investigation	Rationale
Haemoglobin	Anaemia may delay healing
White cell count	Infection
Platelet count	Thrombocytopenia
Erythrocyte sedimentation rate; C reactive protein	Non-specific markers of infection and inflammation; useful in diagnosis and monitoring treatment of infectious or inflammatory ulceration
Urea and creatinine	High urea impairs wound healing. Renal function important when using antibiotics
Albumin	Protein loss delays healing
Glucose, haemoglobin A_{1c}	Diabetes mellitus
Markers of autoimmune disease (such as rheumatoid factor, antinuclear antibodies, anticardiolipin antibodies, lupus anticoagulant)	Indicative of rheumatoid disease, systemic lupus erythematosus, and other connective tissue disorders
Cryoglobulins, cryofibrinogens, prothrombin time, partial thromboplastin time	Haematological disease
Deficiency or defect of antithrombin III, protein C, protein S, factor V Leiden	Vascular thrombosis
Haemoglobinopathy screen	Sickle cell anaemia, thalassaemia
HIV status	Kaposi's sarcoma
Serum protein electrophoresis; Bence-Jones proteins	Myeloma
Urine analysis	Useful in connective tissue disease
Wound swab	Not routine; all ulcers colonised (not the same as infection); swab only when clinical signs of infection

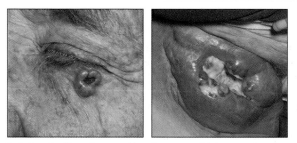

Left: Basal cell carcinoma with rolled edges. Right: Lymphoma presenting as groin ulceration

Site of wound and type of ulcer

Site	Type of ulcer
Gaiter area of the leg	Venous ulcer
Sacrum, greater trochanter, heel	Pressure ulcer
Dorsum of the foot	Arterial or vasculitic ulcer
Shin	Necrobiosis lipoidica
Lateral malleolus	Venous, arterial, or pressure ulcer or hydroxyurea induced ulceration
Plantar and lateral aspect of foot and toes	Diabetic ulcer
Sun exposed areas	Basal cell carcinoma; squamous cell carcinoma

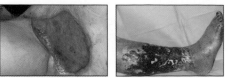

Left: Healthy granulation tissue in a hidradenitis suppurativa excision wound. Right: Unhealthy granulation tissue in a venous leg ulcer

fibrinous tissue (see next article in this series). This tissue is avascular, and healing will proceed only when it is removed. This can be done with a scalpel at the bedside.

The type of tissue at the base of the wound will provide useful information relating to expectation of total healing time and the risk of complications—for example, bone at the base may suggest osteomyelitis and delayed or non-healing.

Necrotic tissue, slough, and eschar

The wound bed may be covered with necrotic tissue (non-viable tissue due to reduced blood supply), slough (dead tissue, usually cream or yellow in colour), or eschar (dry, black, hard necrotic tissue). Such tissue impedes healing. Necrotic tissue and slough may be quantified as excessive (+++), moderate (++), minimal (+), or absent (−).

Since necrotic tissue can also harbour pathogenic organisms, removal of such tissue helps to prevent wound infection. Necrotic tissue and slough should be debrided with a scalpel so that the wound bed can be accurately assessed and facilitate healing. Eschar may be adherent to the wound bed, making debridement with a scalpel difficult. Further debridement, as part of wound management, may be required using other techniques.

Types of debridement

Sharp—At the bedside (using scalpel or curette)
Surgical—In the operating theatre
Autolytic—Facilitation of the body's own mechanism of debridement with appropriate dressings
Biological—Larval (maggot) therapy
Enzymatic—Not widely used; pawpaw (papaya) or banana skin used in developing countries
Mechanical—Wet-to-dry dressings (not widely used in the UK)

Depth

Accurate methods for measuring wound depth are not practical or available in routine clinical practice. However, approximate measurements of greatest depth should be taken to assess wound progress. Undermining of the edge of the wound must be identified by digital examination or use of a probe. The depth and extent of sinuses and fistulas should be identified. Undermining areas and sinuses should be packed with an appropriate dressing to facilitate healing. Undermining wounds and sinuses with narrow necks that are difficult to dress may be amenable to be laid open at the bedside to facilitate drainage and dressing. Wounds associated with multiple sinuses or fistulas should be referred for specialist surgical intervention.

Surrounding skin

Cellulitis associated with wounds should be treated with systemic antibiotics. Eczematous changes may need treatment with potent topical steroid preparations. Maceration of the surrounding skin is often a sign of inability of the dressing to control the wound exudate, which may respond to more frequent dressing changes or change in dressing type. Callus surrounding and sometimes covering neuropathic foot ulcers (for example, in diabetic patients) must be debrided to (a) visualise the wound, (b) eliminate potential source of infection, and (c) remove areas close to the wound subject to abnormal pressure that would otherwise cause enlargement of the wound. This can be done at the bedside.

Infection

All open wounds are colonised. Bacteriological culture is indicated only if clinical signs of infection are present or if

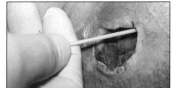

Bone at the base of a wound may suggest a protracted healing time and the possibility of underlying osteomyelitis

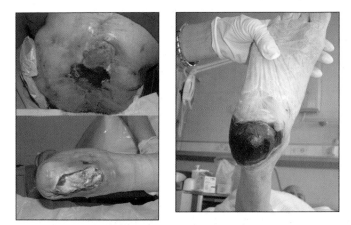

Top: Necrotic tissue (black areas) in a pressure ulcer. Bottom: Slough at the base of a pressure ulcer. Right: Eschar covering a heel pressure ulcer

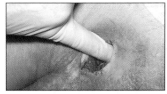

Left: Digital examination of a wound. Right: Examining a wound with a probe

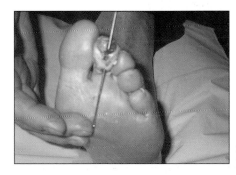

Fistula in a diabetic foot ulcer

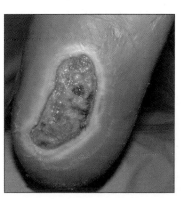

Maceration of the skin surrounding a diabetic foot ulcer

infection control issues (such as methicillin resistant staphylococcus aureus (MRSA)) need to be considered. The classic signs of infection are heat, redness, swelling, and pain. Additional signs of wound infection include increased exudate, delayed healing, contact bleeding, odour, and abnormal granulation tissue. Treatment with antimicrobials should be guided by microbiological results and local resistance patterns.

Pain

Pain is a characteristic feature of many healing and non-healing wounds. Pain can be caused by both nociceptive and neuropathic stimuli. Intermittent pain is often related to dressing removal or recent application of new dressings and may necessitate the use of analgesia before the dressing is changed. Constant pain may arise as a result of the underlying condition, such as ischaemia, neuropathy, tissue oedema, chronic tissue damage (for example, lipodermatosclerosis), infection, or scarring (for example, atrophie blanche). The nature and type of pain should be identified and treated appropriately. Pain assessment tools can help to assess the nature and severity of pain. With recalcitrant pain, or pain that is difficult to control, consider referral to a local pain team.

Non-healing wounds

Non-healing wounds have traditionally been defined as those that fail to progress through an orderly sequence of repair in a timely fashion. Such wounds are sometimes thought of as being caused by neglect, incompetence, misdiagnosis, or inappropriate treatment strategies. However, some wounds are resistant to all efforts of treatment aimed at healing, and alternative end points should be considered; measures aimed at improving the quality of life will be paramount in these instances.

Quality of life

Several studies have shown that patients with non-healing wounds have a decreased quality of life. Reasons for this include the frequency and regularity of dressing changes, which affect daily routine; a feeling of continued fatigue due to lack of sleep; restricted mobility; pain; odour; wound infection; and the physical and psychological effects of polypharmacy. The loss of independence associated with functional decline can lead to changes, sometimes subtle, in overall health and wellbeing. These changes include altered eating habits, depression, social isolation, and a gradual reduction in activity levels. Many patients with non-healing wounds complain of difficulties with emotions, finances, physical health, daily activities, friendships, and leisure pursuits.

Quality of life is not always related to healing of the wound. It may be clear from the outset that wounds in some patients will be unlikely to heal. In such patients control of symptoms and signs outlined above—particularly odour, exudate, and pain—may improve the individual's quality of life. Additionally, optimal chronic wound management will lead to a reduction in the frequency of dressing changes, further enhancing quality of life. In a minority of instances, seemingly drastic measures—such as amputation in a person with chronic leg ulceration—may need to be considered when the quality of life is severely affected by the non-healing wound and its complications.

The drawing on page 1 is adapted from one provided by Wendy Tyrrell, School of Health and Social Sciences, University of Wales Institute, Cardiff.

Wound exudate

- Wound exudate may be serous, serosanguinous, or sanguinous
- The quantity of exudate is usually classified as heavy (+++ (dressing soaked)), medium (++ (dressing wet)), or minimal (+ (dressing dry))
- Excessive exudate may be due to wound infection or gross oedema in the wound area and may complicate wound healing
- The exudate should be controlled with the use of dressings appropriate for the level of exudate and any infection treated
- Barrier films applied to the surrounding skin help to prevent further maceration (see the ninth article in the series)
- The oedematous leg should be raised when the patient is seated

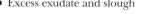

The causes of malodorous wounds include infection and the presence of necrotic tissue. Infection should be treated with antibiotics. Odour associated with necrotic tissue may be reduced by removal of the necrotic tissue or use of agents impregnated with antiseptics or charcoal. Treatment with topical metronidazole and use of odour absorbing dressings may help to reduce odour from fungating malignant wounds. Larval therapy may also be helpful in the debridement of malodorous tissue

Clinical features of non-healing wounds

- Absence of healthy granulation tissue
- Presence of necrotic and unhealthy tissue in the wound bed
- Excess exudate and slough
- Lack of adequate blood supply
- Failure of re-epithelialisation
- Cyclical or persistent pain
- Recurrent breakdown of wound
- Clinical or subclinical infection

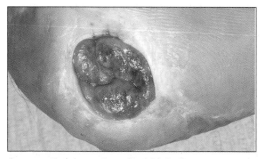

Overgranulation may be a sign of infection or non-healing

Further reading

- Lazarus GS, Cooper DM, Knighton DR, Margolis DJ, Pecoraro RE, Rodeheaver G, et al. Definitions and guidelines for assessment of wounds and evaluation of healing. *Arch Dermatol* 1994;130:489-93.
- Izadi K, Ganchi P. Chronic wounds. *Clin Plast Surg* 2005;32:209-22.
- Falanga V, Phillips TJ, Harding KG, Moy RL, Peerson LJ, eds. *Text atlas of wound management*. London: Martin Dunitz, 2000.

Competing interests: KGH's unit receives income from many commercial companies for research and education, and for advice. It does not support one company's products over another.

2 Venous and arterial leg ulcers

Joseph E Grey, Stuart Enoch, Keith G Harding

Venous ulceration

Venous leg ulceration is due to sustained venous hypertension, which results from chronic venous insufficiency. In the normal venous system, pressure decreases with exercise as a result of the action of the calf muscle pump. When the muscles relax, the valves in the perforating veins connecting the superficial to the deep venous circulation prevent reflux and the pressure remains low. The venous pressure remains high, however, in a system where the valves are incompetent.

Up to 10% of the population in Europe and North America has valvular incompetence, with 0.2% developing venous ulceration. Forty to fifty per cent of venous ulcers are due to superficial venous insufficiency and/or perforating vein incompetence alone with a normal deep venous system.

There are many risk factors for venous ulceration. Recurrent venous ulceration occurs in up to 70% of those at risk. Many venous ulcers are painful, so appropriate pain relief and advice should be given.

Risk factors for venous ulceration

Direct risk factors
- Varicose veins
- Deep vein thrombosis
- Chronic venous insufficiency
- Poor calf muscle function
- Arterio-venous fistulae
- Obesity
- History of leg fracture

Indirect risk factors
- All risk factors leading to deep vein thrombosis including protein-C, protein-S, and anti-thrombin III deficiency
- Family history of varicose veins
- A history of minor trauma prior to the development of ulceration may also be identified

Examination

Ninety five per cent of venous ulceration is in the gaiter area of the leg, characteristically around the malleoli. Ulceration may be discrete or circumferential. The ulcer bed is often covered with a fibrinous layer mixed with granulation tissue, surrounded by an irregular, gently sloping edge. Ulcers occurring above the mid-calf or on the foot are likely to have other origins.

Pitting oedema is often present and may predate the ulcer. It is often worse towards the end of the day. Extravasation of erythrocytes into the skin occurs, resulting in the deposition of haemosiderin within macrophages, which stimulates melanin production, pigmenting the skin brown. In long term venous insufficiency, lipodermatosclerosis occurs. This is characterised

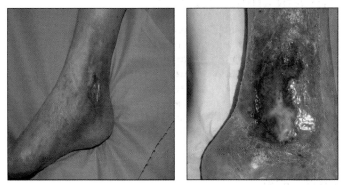

Typical venous leg ulcer over the medial malleolus (left) and venous leg ulcer over malleolus with a fibrinous base (right)

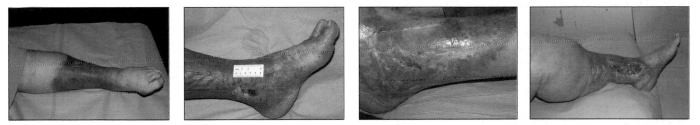

From left to right: Haemosiderin associated with a venous leg ulcer; lipodermatosclerosis; venous leg ulcer in area of atrophie blanche; venous leg ulcer with severe "champagne bottle" deformity of the leg

by the dermis and subcutaneous tissue becoming indurated and fibrosed with the lack of pitting oedema; the skin also becomes atrophic, loses sweat glands and hair follicles, and becomes variably pigmented (ranging from hypopigmented to hyperpigmented). Severe lipodermatosclerosis may lead to atrophie blanche—white fibrotic areas with low blood flow. Lipodermatosclerosis often precedes venous ulceration. As a result of lipodermatosclerosis, a rigid woody hardness often develops, which at its worst may result in the leg resembling an "inverted champagne bottle." Venous eczema (erythema, scaling, weeping, and itching) is also common and is distinct from cellulitis.

Features of venous eczema and cellulitis

Venous eczema	Cellulitis
Red, warm, painful, and tender to touch	Red, warm, painful, and tender to touch
Usually chronic	Insidious (usually develops over 24-72 hours)
Diffuse and poorly demarcated	Usually well demarcated
Increase in exudate	No increase in exudate
Itchy	Not itchy
Scaly	Not scaly
Treated with topical steroids	Treated with systemic antibiotics

Management

Compression is the mainstay of venous ulcer management (see also 11th article in this series). Graded compression, with greatest pressure (about 40 mm Hg) at the ankle, tapering off to lower pressure (about 18 mm Hg) below the knee, increases the limb hydrostatic pressure and concomitantly reduces the superficial venous pressure. Various compression bandage systems are used. These include the single and multilayer elastic banadage system, short stretch bandage, and elasticated tubular bandages (for example, Tubigrip). Compression with pneumatic devices (for example, Flowtron) has been used to promote healing of venous ulcers in patients with oedematous legs.

Patients should be warned to remove the compression if they notice any side effects (such as numbness, tingling, pain, and dusky toes) and seek advice.

Sharp debridement of non-viable tissue may expedite healing of venous ulcers and can be done in the primary care setting. Surgery is normally indicated to correct superficial venous disease in an attempt to prevent ulcers from recurring. Shave therapy (excision of the whole ulcer) followed by skin grafting, or skin grafting alone, may be useful in patients where other treatments have failed.

Venous leg ulcers often become infected (see 10th article in this series for how to detect signs of infection). The most common organisms include *Staphylococcus aureus*, *Pseudomonas aeruginosa*, and β-haemolytic streptococci. Initially, these should be treated empirically (with broad spectrum penicillin or macrolide or quinolone antibiotics) until definitive culture and sensitivities are available. Infection should be treated with a two week course of antibiotics. Topical antibiotics should be avoided owing to the risk of increasing bacterial resistance and contact dermatitis. Associated venous eczema should be treated with topical steroids and emollients. The eczema may be secondarily infected and require systemic antibiotic therapy.

Once the venous ulcer has healed, it is essential that patients follow simple advice aimed at preventing the recurrence of the ulcer: this includes wearing compression stockings, skin care, leg elevation, calf exercises, and adopting a suitable diet. The reported annual recurrence rate of venous ulcers (20%) is strongly influenced by patient adherence. Local "leg clubs"(www.legclub.org) may help to reduce this rate.

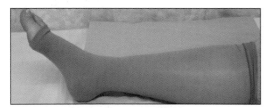

Compression stocking

Arterial ulceration

Arterial ulceration is due to a reduced arterial blood supply to the lower limb. The most common cause is atherosclerotic disease of the medium and large sized arteries. Other causes include diabetes, thromboangiitis, vasculitis, pyoderma gangrenosum, thalassaemia, and sickle cell disease, some of which may predispose to the formation of atheroma. Further damage to the arterial system occurs with concurrent hypertension through damage of the intimal layer of the artery. The reduction in arterial blood supply results in tissue hypoxia and tissue damage. Thrombotic and atheroembolic episodes may contribute to tissue damage and ulcer formation.

> Unna's boot, a wet zinc oxide bandage applied from toes to knee and covered with elastic compression bandage, is commonly used in the United States. The surrounding skin, however, can develop contact dermatitis, and this type of bandaging may fail to control high levels of exudate from the ulcer

---

Choice of dressing

- Dressing choice will reflect the nature of the ulcer (see ninth article in this series)
- The leg should always be raised when a patient is seated
- Patients should be encouraged, however, to remain active provided they are wearing some form of compression system

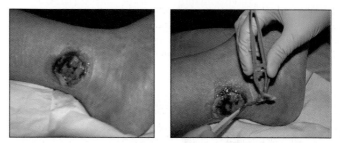

Unhealthy venous leg ulcer before debridement (left) and sharp debridement of venous leg ulcer (right)

Compression stockings

Class	Pressure at ankle (mm Hg)	Indication
I	14-17	Mild varicose veins
II	18-24	Prevention of recurrence of venous ulcers on narrow legs and in slim patients and for mild oedema
III	25-35	Chronic venous insufficiency and oedema, and large heavy legs

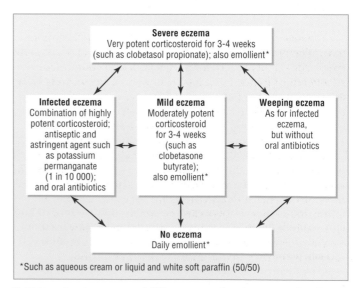

Guidelines for management of different categories of venous eczema. Arrows indicate direction of possible change in condition of eczema

---

> Arterial ulceration often occurs after seemingly trivial trauma or as the result of localised pressure

Peripheral vascular disease is most common in men older than 45 and women older than 55, and patients may have a family history of premature atherosclerotic disease. Modifiable risk factors for peripheral vascular disease include smoking, hyperlipidaemia, hypertension, diabetes, and obesity, with associated decreased activity. Patients may also have a history of generalised vascular problems, such as myocardial infarction, angina, stroke, and intermittent claudication.

Examination

Arterial ulceration typically occurs over the toes, heels, and bony prominences of the foot. The ulcer appears "punched out," with well demarcated edges and a pale, non-granulating, often necrotic base. The surrounding skin may exhibit dusky erythema and may be cool to touch, hairless, thin, and brittle, with a shiny texture. The toenails thicken and become opaque and may be lost. Gangrene of the extremities may also occur. Examination of the arterial system may show a decreased or absent pulse in the dorsalis pedis and posterior tibial arteries. There may be bruits in the proximal leg arteries, indicating the presence of atherosclerosis.

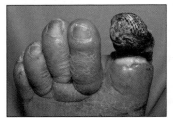
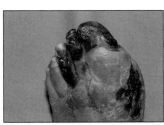
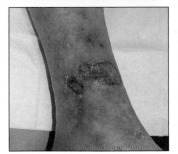

Top left: Dry gangrene of great toe in a patient with peripheral vascular disease with line of demarcation covered with slough. Top right: Wet gangrene of forefoot and toes in a patient with arterial disease, with soft tissue swelling due to infection. Left: Arterial ulcer over lower leg, with associated skin changes typical of arterial disease

Patients with arterial ulcers have a reduced capillary refill time. With normal capillary refill, after compression of the great toe or dorsum of the foot for a few seconds, the skin colour should return to normal in less than two to three seconds. Delay in return of the normal colour is indicative of vascular compromise. A delay of more than 10 to 15 seconds in return of colour after raising an ischaemic leg to 45 degrees for one minute (Buerger's test) indicates vascular compromise.

The ankle brachial pressure index is helpful in identifying peripheral vascular disease in the absence of non-compressible vessels resulting from vessel calcification (for example, diabetes) or tissue oedema. A duplex ultrasound scan will give further information—on arterial occlusion, stenosis, and areas of diffuse and continuous atheromatous disease. Arteriography is the ideal investigation in preoperative planning, allowing direct assessment of the vascular anatomy of the lower limb.

Management

Increasing the peripheral blood flow by, for example, reconstructive surgery (for diffuse disease) or angioplasty (for localised stenosis) is the intervention most likely to affect the healing process in arterial ulceration. Operative indications for chronic ischaemia include non-healing ulceration, gangrene, rest pain, and progression of disabling claudication.

Pain with arterial ulceration

- Pain may be present at rest and may be alleviated by hanging the foot over the side of the bed or sleeping in a chair
- Pain usually begins distal to the obstruction, moving proximally as ischaemia progresses
- The ulcer itself is often painful

Features of venous and arterial ulcers

	Venous	Arterial
History	History of varicose veins, deep vein thrombosis, venous insufficiency or venous incompetence	History suggestive of peripheral arterial disease, intermittent claudication, and/or rest pain
Classic site	Over the medial gaiter region of the leg	Usually over the toes, foot, and ankle
Edges	Sloping	Punched out
Wound bed	Often covered with slough	Often covered with varying degrees of slough and necrotic tissue
Exudate level	Usually high	Usually low
Pain	Pain not severe unless associated with excessive oedema or infection	Pain, even without infection
Oedema	Usually associated with limb oedema	Oedema not common
Associated features	Venous eczema, lipodermatosclerosis, atrophie blanche, haemosiderosis	Trophic changes; gangrene may be present
Treatment	Compression is mainstay	Appropriate surgery for arterial insufficiency; drugs of limited value

Interpreting ankle brachial pressure index

Index	Signs and symptoms	Severity of disease	Action
≥0.7-1	Mild intermittent claudication, or no symptoms	Mild arterial disease	Reduce risk factors and change lifestyle: stop smoking, maintain weight, exercise regularly, consider antiplatelet agent
0.7-0.5	Varying degrees of intermittent claudication	Mild to moderate arterial disease	As for index ≥0.7-1, plus referral to outpatient vascular specialist and possible arterial imaging (duplex scan and/or angiogram)
0.5-0.3	Severe intermittent claudication and rest pain	Severe arterial disease	As for index ≥0.7-1, plus urgent referral to vascular specialist and possible arterial imaging (duplex scan and/or angiogram)
≤0.3 or ankle systolic pressure <50 mm Hg	Critical ischaemia (rest pain >2 weeks) with or without tissue loss (ulcer, gangrene)	Severe arterial disease; risk of losing limb	Urgent referral to vascular emergency on-call team and possible surgical or radiological intervention

An index of 1 to 1.1 is considered to be normal. The data in the table should be used as an adjunct to the clinical findings. Erroneous readings may be the result of incompressible arteries secondary to presence of calcification or presence of tissue oedema. Patients may present with an arterial ulcer even with a normal index. Patients may present with an acutely ischaemic limb either due to an embolus or a thrombus ("acute on chronic" ischaemia) and should be referred as an emergency to a vascular specialist or emergency department for urgent intervention to prevent imminent limb loss.

The patient should stop smoking, and control of diabetes, hypertension, and hyperlipidaemia should be optimised. Patients may find benefits from sleeping in a bed raised at the head end. Patients should follow simple advice on foot and leg care. Walking is beneficial.

Infection can cause rapid deterioration in an arterial ulcer, and treatment with systemic antibiotics (along the lines for venous ulceration outlined above) should be started. Patients with rest pain or worsening claudication, or both, and a non-healing ulcer should be referred to a vascular surgeon; opioid analgesia may be necessary during the wait for surgery. It is not appropriate to debride arterial ulcers as this may promote further ischaemia and lead to the formation of a larger ulcer.

Choice of wound dressings will be dictated by the nature of the wound. Vasoconstrictive drugs such as non-selective β blockers should be avoided. (See chapter 11 for more information on drug treatment.)

Ulceration of mixed aetiology is not uncommon: patients may have a combination of venous and arterial diseases, resulting in ulcers of mixed aetiologies, which will limit the degree of compression (if any) that can be used.

Guidelines for patients on protecting lower limbs and feet

- Examine the feet daily for broken skin, blisters, swelling, or redness
- Report worsening symptoms—for example, decreasing walking distance, pain at rest, pain at night, changes in skin colour
- Keep the skin moist with, for example, 50/50 white soft paraffin and liquid paraffin mix
- Never walk barefoot
- Ensure shoes are well fitting and free of friction and pressure points; check them for foreign objects (such as stones) before wearing; and avoid open toed sandals and pointed shoes
- Give up smoking
- Take regular exercise within limits of pain and tolerance

Further reading

- Simon DA, Dix FP, McCollum CN. Management of venous leg ulcers. *BMJ* 2004;328:1358-62.
- Barwell JR, Davies CE, Deacon J, Harvey K, Minor J, Sassano A, et al. Comparison of surgery and compression with compression alone in chronic venous ulceration (ESCHAR study): randomised controlled trial. *Lancet* 2004;363:1854-9.
- Cullum N, Nelson EA, Fletcher AW, Sheldon TA. Compression for venous leg ulcers. *Cochrane Database Syst Rev* 2001;(2):CD000265.
- Williams DT, Enoch S, Miller DR, Harris K, Price PE, Harding KG. The effect of sharp debridement using curette on recalcitrant non-healing venous leg ulcers: a concurrently controlled prospective cohort study. *Wound Rep Regen* 2005;13:131-7.
- Morris PJ, Malt RA. *Oxford textbook of surgery.* 2nd ed. Oxford: Oxford University Press, 2001.
- Burnand KG, Young AE, Lucas JD, Rowlands B, Scholefield J. *The new Aird's companion in surgical studies.* 2nd ed. Edinburgh: Elsevier Churchill Livingstone, 2005.
- Nelson EA, Bell-Syer SE, Cullum NA. Compression for preventing recurrence of venous ulcers. *Cochrane Database Syst Rev* 2000;(4):CD002303.
- Gohel MS, Barwell JR, Earnshaw JJ, Heather BP, Mitchell DC, Whyman MR, et al. Randomized clinical trial of compression plus surgery versus compression alone in chronic venous ulceration (ESCHAR study)—haemodynamic and anatomical changes. *Br J Surg* 2005;92:291-7.

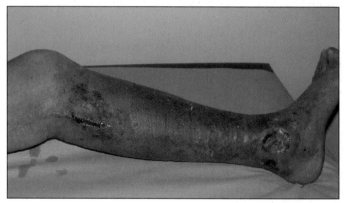

Ulcer over medial malleolus of mixed arterial and venous aetiology, with lipodermatosclerosis and breakdown of scar over saphenous vein harvesting site (for cardiac bypass grafting)

The table on interpreting the ankle brachial pressure index is adapted from Beard JD, Gaines PA, eds. *Vascular and endovascular surgery.* 3rd ed. London: WB Saunders, 2005.

3 Diabetic foot ulcers

Michael E Edmonds, A V M Foster

Diabetic foot ulcers can be divided into two groups: those in neuropathic feet (so called neuropathic ulcers) and those in feet with ischaemia often associated with neuropathy (so called neuroischaemic ulcers). The neuropathic foot is warm and well perfused with palpable pulses; sweating is diminished, and the skin may be dry and prone to fissuring. The neuroischaemic foot is a cool, pulseless foot; the skin is thin, shiny, and without hair. There is also atrophy of the subcutaneous tissue, and intermittent claudication and rest pain may be absent because of neuropathy.

The crucial difference between the two types of feet is the absence or presence of ischaemia. The presence of ischaemia may be confirmed by a pressure index (ankle brachial pressure index < 1). As many diabetic patients have medial arterial calcification, giving an artificially raised ankle systolic pressure, it is also important to examine the Doppler arterial waveform. The normal waveform is pulsatile with a positive forward flow in systole followed by a short reverse flow and a further forward flow in diastole, but in the presence of arterial narrowing the waveform shows a reduced forward flow and is described as "damped."

Neuropathic foot ulcer

Neuropathic ulcers usually occur on the plantar aspect of the foot under the metatarsal heads or on the plantar aspects of the toes.

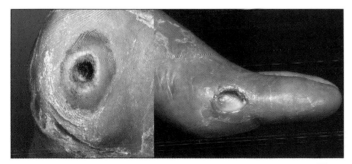

Left: Neuropathic foot with plantar ulcer surrounded by callus. Right: Ulcer over medial aspect of first metatarsophalangeal joint of neuroischaemic foot

The most common cause of ulceration is repetitive mechanical forces of gait, which lead to callus, the most important preulcerative lesion in the neuropathic foot. If allowed to become too thick, the callus will press on the soft tissues underneath and cause ulceration. A layer of whitish, macerated, moist tissue found under the surface of the callus indicates that the foot is close to ulceration, and urgent removal of the callus is necessary. If the callus is not removed, inflammatory autolysis and haematomas develop under the callus. This leads to tissue necrosis, resulting in a small cavity filled with serous fluid giving the appearance of a blister under the callus. Removal of the callus reveals an ulcer.

A foot ulcer is a sign of systemic disease and should never be regarded as trivial

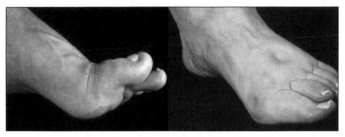

Left: Neuropathic foot with prominent metatarsal heads and pressure points over the plantar forefoot. Right: Neuroischaemic foot showing pitting oedema secondary to cardiac failure, and hallux valgus and erythema from pressure from tight shoe on medial aspect of first metatarsophalangeal joint

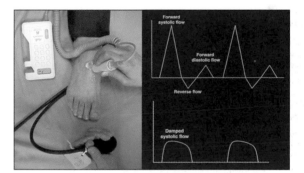

Left: Hand held Doppler used with sphygmomanometer to measure ankle systolic pressure. Right: Doppler waveform from normal foot showing normal triphasic pattern (top) and from neuroischaemic foot showing damped pattern (bottom)

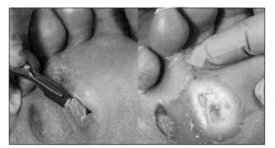

Left: Callus removal by sharp debridement. Right: Whitish, macerated, moist tissue under surface of callus, indicating imminent ulceration

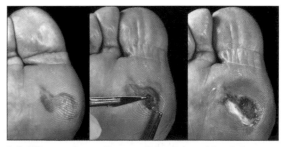

Left: Blister under a callus over first metatarsal head. Centre: The roof of the blister is grasped in forceps and cut away, together with associated callus. Right: Ulcer is revealed underneath

Neuroischaemic foot ulcer

Neuroischaemic ulcers are often seen on the margins of the foot, especially on the medial surface of the first metatarsophalangeal joint and over the lateral aspect of the fifth metatarsophalangeal joint. They also develop on the tips of the toes and beneath any toe nails if these become overly thick.

The classic sign of preulceration in the neuroischaemic foot is a red mark on the skin, often precipitated by tight shoes or a slip-on shoe, leading to frictional forces on the vulnerable margins of the foot.

The first sign of ischaemic ulceration is a superficial blister, usually secondary to friction. It then develops into a shallow ulcer with a base of sparse pale granulation tissue or yellowish closely adherent slough.

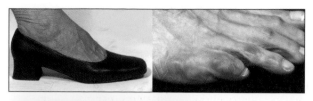
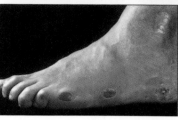

Top: Shoe with no proper fastening and with a narrow toe box (left); red marks on toes after wearing unsuitable shoes (right). Left: New ischaemic ulcers resulting from bullae on lateral margin of foot

Management

Wound control

In the neuropathic foot, all callus surrounding the ulcer is removed with a scalpel, together with slough and non-viable tissue. It is always important to probe the ulcer as this may reveal a sinus extending to bone (suggesting osteomyelitis) or undermining of the edges where the probe can be passed from the ulcer underneath surrounding intact skin.

In the neuroischaemic foot, slough and dried necrotic material should be removed from the ulcer by sharp debridement. Debridement should be cautious if the foot is very ischaemic (pressure index < 0.5) as it is essential not to damage viable tissue.

Some ischaemic ulcers develop a halo of thin glassy callus that dries out, becomes hard, and curls up. These areas need to be smoothed off as they can catch on dressings and cause trauma to underlying tissue. If a subungual ulcer is suspected, the nail should be cut back very gently or layers of nail pared away, to expose and drain the ulcer. Maggot therapy is sometimes used in debridement, especially with neuroischaemic ulcers.

Vacuum assisted closure may be used to achieve closure of diabetic foot ulcers and wounds that have been debrided. This technique is increasingly used to treat postoperative wounds in a diabetic ischaemic foot, especially when revasularisation is not possible.

Mechanical control

In neuropathic feet the overall aim is to redistribute plantar pressures, wheareas in neuroischaemic feet it is to protect the vulnerable margins of the foot. Semicompressed adhesive felt padding may be used to divert pressure, especially from small ulcers in neuropathic feet. The most efficient way to redistribute plantar pressure is to use a total contact cast (treatment of choice for indolent neuropathic ulcers), a prefabricated cast such as Aircast, or a Scotchcast boot.

If casting techniques are not available, temporary shoes with a cushioning insole can be supplied. When the neuropathic ulcer has healed, the patient should be fitted with a cradled insole and bespoke shoes to prevent recurrence. Occasionally, extra-deep, "off the shelf" orthopaedic shoes with flat cushioning insoles may suffice in the absence of areas of very high pressure.

As ulcers in neuroischaemic feet usually develop around the margins of the foot, a shoe bought from a high street shop may be adequate provided that the shoe is sufficiently long, broad, and deep and fastens with a lace or strap high on the foot. Alternatively, a Scotchcast boot or a wide-fitting, off the shelf shoe may be suitable.

The ulcer should be cleansed and dressed with an appropriate dressing (see chapter 9 in this series)

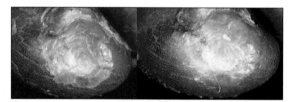

Left: Ischaemic ulcer with halo of thin glassy callus. Right: The halo has been cut away without causing trauma

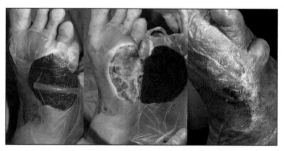

Left: Vacuum assisted pump sponge attached to plantar aspect of foot. Centre: Pump sponge being removed from foot. Right: Healed wound

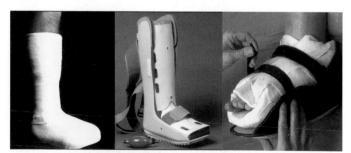

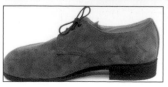

Top (left to right): Total contact cast; Aircast prefabricated cast; Scotchcast boot. Left: A suitable shoe bought in the high street may be sufficiently roomy to avoid pressure

Pressure ulcer in the diabetic foot

All patients with neuropathic or neuroischaemic feet are at risk of pressure ulcers, especially of the heel. Pressure over heel ulcers can be off-loaded by "pressure relief ankle foot orthoses." This orthosis is a ready-made device that has a washable fleece liner with an aluminium and polypropylene adjustable frame and a non-slip, neoprene base for walking. It is used to relieve pressure over the posterior aspect of the heel and maintain the ankle joint in a suitable position, thus preventing pressure ulceration, aiding healing, and preventing deformity.

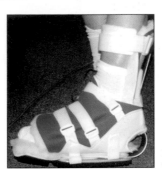

Pressure relief ankle/foot orthosis for use with heel ulcers

Vascular control

If an ischaemic ulcer has not shown progress in healing despite optimum treatment, then it may be possible to do duplex ultrasound and angiography. This should be done if any or all of the following are present:

- An ankle brachial pressure index of <0.5 or a damped Doppler waveform
- A transcutaneous oxygen (reflecting local arterial perfusion pressure) of <30 mm Hg
- A toe pressure of <30 mm Hg.

Duplex ultrasound and angiography may show areas of stenoses or occlusions suitable for angioplasty. If lesions are too extensive for angioplasty, then arterial bypass may be considered.

Another manifestation of ischaemia is dry gangrene, particularly in a toe. Dry gangrene usually results from severe ischaemia secondary to poor tissue perfusion from atherosclerotic narrowing of the arteries of the leg. Ideally, the ischaemic foot should be revascularised and the digital necrosis be removed surgically, but if revascularisation is not possible, the gangrenous parts of the toes may be allowed to "autoamputate" (drop off naturally).

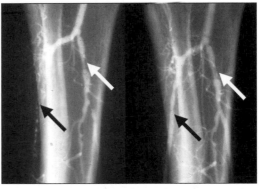

Left: Angiogram showing occlusion of anterior tibial artery and stenosis of tibioperoneal trunk. Right: Post-angioplasty anterior tibial flow has been restored and tibioperoneal stenosis dilated

Microbiological control

When an ulcer is present, there is a clear entrance for invading bacteria. Infection can range from local infection of the ulcer to wet gangrene. Only half of infection episodes show signs of infection. In the presence of neuropathy and ischaemia, the inflammatory response is impaired and early signs of infection may be subtle.

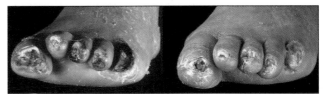

Left: Necrotic fifth toe and necrotic apices of the first, third, and fourth toes undergoing podiatric debridement. Right: Autoamputation six weeks later, after regular debridement

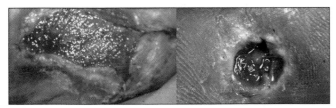

Left: Increased friable granulation tissue. Right: Base of ulcer has areas of yellowish to grey tissue

Deep swab and tissue samples (not surface callus) should be sent for culture without delay and wide spectrum antibiotics given to cover Gram positive, Gram negative, and anaerobic bacteria. Urgent surgical intervention is needed in certain circumstances.

Local signs of wound infection

- Granulation tissue becomes increasingly friable
- Base of the ulcer becomes moist and changes from healthy pink granulations to yellowish or grey tissue
- Discharge changes from clear to purulent
- Unpleasant odour is present

Indications for urgent surgical intervention

- Large area of infected sloughy tissue
- Localised fluctuance and expression of pus
- Crepitus with gas in the soft tissues on x ray examination
- Purplish discoloration of the skin, indicating subcutaneous necrosis

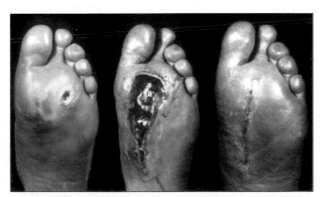

Left: Deep ulcer with subcutaneous sloughing visible. Centre: Extent of debridement necessary to remove all necrotic tissue down to healthy bleeding tissue. Right: Wound has healed at 10 weeks

ABC of wound healing

In neuropathic feet, gangrene is almost invariably wet and is caused by infection of a digital, metatarsal, or heel ulcer that leads to a septic vasculitis of the digital and small arteries of the foot. The walls of these arteries are infiltrated by polymorphs, leading to occlusion of the lumen by septic thrombus. Wet gangrene may need surgical intervention.

Wet gangrene caused by septic vasculitis can also occur in neuroischaemic feet, although reduced arterial perfusion due to atherosclerotic occlusive disease is an important predisposing factor. Gangrenous tissue should be surgically removed and the foot revascularised if possible.

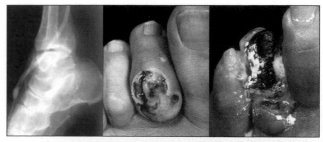

Left: Vein bypass seen passing across ankle to the dorsalis pedis artery. Centre: Infected ulcer with cellulitis. Right: Wet necrosis from infected toe ulcer

Metabolic control

Wound healing and neutrophil function is impaired by hyperglycaemia, so tight glycaemic control is essential. Patients with type 2 diabetes suboptimally controlled with oral hypoglycaemic drugs should be prescribed insulin. Hyperlipidaemia and hypertension should be treated. Patients should stop smoking. Those with neuroischaemic ulcers should take statins and antiplatelets. Diabetic patients with peripheral vascular disease may also benefit from an angiotensin converting enzyme inhibitor to prevent further vascular episodes.

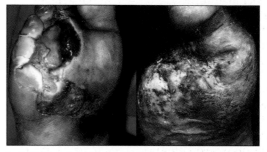

Left: Plantar view of infection after puncture wound that led to wet necrosis of the forefoot requiring amputation of four toes and their adjoining metatarsal heads. Right: Full healing of the large post-surgical tissue defect took six months

Education

Patients who have lost protective pain sensation need advice on how to protect their feet from mechanical, thermal, and chemical trauma. Patients should be instructed on the principles of ulcer care with emphasis on the importance of rest, footwear, regular dressings, and frequent observation for signs of infection. They should be taught the four danger signs: swelling, pain, colour change, and breaks in the skin.

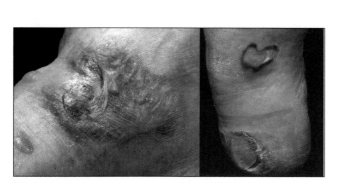

Left: Thermal trauma from convection heater. Right: Ulceration after use of foot spa

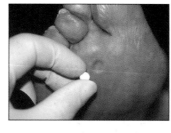

Oral hypoglycaemic agent found within the patient's shoe at annual review

Members of the multidisciplinary team

- Physician
- Podiatrist
- Specialist nurse
- Orthotist
- Dietitian
- Radiologist
- Vascular surgeon
- Orthopaedic surgeon

Further reading

- Edmonds M, Foster AVM, Sanders L. *A practical manual of diabetic foot care.* Oxford: Blackwell Science, 2004.
- Bowker JH, Pfeifer MA, eds. *Levin and O'Neal's the diabetic foot.* 6th ed. St Louis: Mosby, 2001.
- Boulton AJM, Connor H, Cavanagh PR, eds. *The foot in diabetes.* 3rd ed. Chichester: Wiley, 2000.
- The International Working Group on the Diabetic Foot. *International consensus on the diabetic foot.* 2003 (www.iwgdf.org/concensus/introduction.htm)
- Veves A, Giurini JM, Logerfo FW, eds. *The diabetic foot. Medical and surgical management.* Totowa, NJ: Humana Press, 2002.
- National Institute for Clinical Excellence. *Type 2 diabetes. Prevention and management of foot problems.* London: NICE, 2004. (www.nice.org.uk/pdf/CG010NICEguideline.pdf)

Successful management of diabetic feet requires the expertise of a multidisciplinary team that provides integrated care, rapid access clinics, early diagnosis, and prompt treatment. Patients will need close follow-up for the rest of their lives

4 Pressure ulcers

Joseph E Grey, Stuart Enoch, Keith G Harding

A pressure ulcer is defined by the European Pressure Ulcer Advisory Panel as an area of localised damage to the skin and underlying tissue caused by pressure, shear, or friction, or a combination of these. Pressure ulcers are caused by a local breakdown of soft tissue as a result of compression between a bony prominence and an external surface.

They usually develop on the lower half of the body: two thirds around the pelvis and a third on the lower limbs, with heel ulceration becoming more common. Elderly people are the most likely group to have pressure ulcers; this is especially true for those older than 70, up to a third of whom will have had surgery for a hip fracture. Those with spinal injuries form another distinct group, in whom the prevalence is 20%-30% one to five years after injury.

Most pressure ulcers arise in hospital, where the prevalence among inpatients is 3%-14%, although it can be as high as 70% in elderly inpatients with orthopaedic problems. The incidence of pressure ulcers in hospitals is 1%-5%. In patients who are confined to bed or to a chair for more than one week, the incidence rises to almost 8%. In long term healthcare facilities 1.5%-25% of patients develop pressure ulcers. Almost a fifth of pressure ulcers develop at home and a further fifth in nursing homes. The prevalence of pressure ulcers in nursing homes is not much higher than in hospitals. Pressure ulceration in elderly patients is associated with a fivefold increase in mortality, and in-hospital mortality in this group is 25%-33%. Estimates of the cost of pressure ulceration to the NHS range from £180m ($318m; €265m) to nearly £2bn a year.

Pathogenesis

The four main factors implicated are interface pressure, shear, friction, and moisture.

When pressure of short duration is relieved, tissues demonstrate reactive hyperaemia, reflecting increased blood flow to the area. However, sustained high pressure leads to decreased capillary blood flow, occlusion of blood vessels and lymphatic vessels, and tissue ischaemia.

These changes are ultimately responsible for necrosis of muscle, subcutaneous tissue, dermis and epidermis, and consequent formation of pressure ulcers. An external pressure of 50 mm Hg may rise to over 200 mm Hg at a bony prominence, leading, with time, to deep tissue destruction, which may not be evident on the surface of the skin. Regular relief from high pressures in the at-risk patient is essential to prevent pressure ulceration.

Shear force is generated by the motion of bone and subcutaneous tissue relative to the skin, which is restrained from moving due to frictional forces (for example, when a seated patient slides down a chair or when the head of a bed is raised more than 30°). In such circumstances the pressure needed to occlude the blood vessels is greatly reduced. In elderly patients, a reduced amount of elastin in the skin predisposes to the adverse effects of shear.

Friction opposes the movement of one surface against another. Frictional forces may lead to the formation of intraepidermal blisters, which in turn lead to superficial skin erosions, initiating or accelerating pressure ulceration. Such

Most pressure ulcers are avoidable

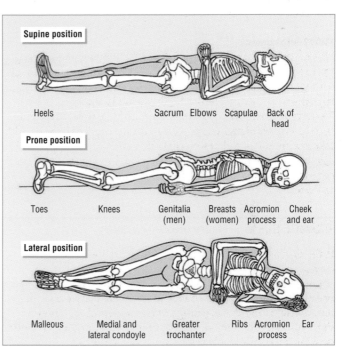

Common sites of pressure ulceration in individuals at risk of ulceration

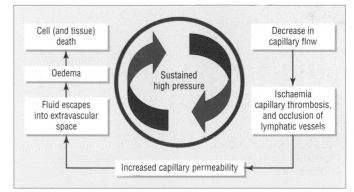

Pathophysiology of pressure ulceration

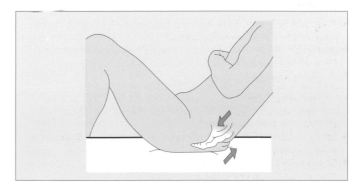

Shear force generated—for example, when a patient slides down a bed

forces occur, for example, when a patient is dragged across a bed sheet or as a result of ill fitting prosthetic devices or footwear.

An excessively moist environment caused, for example, by perspiration, urinary or faecal incontinence, or excessive wound drainage increases the deleterious effects of pressure, friction, and shear. It also causes maceration of the surrounding skin, which compounds these factors. Friction and moisture exert their greatest effects in areas of high pressure: the effects of friction are up to five times worse if moisture is present.

Classification

Among the various classification schemes for pressure ulceration, the one developed by the European Pressure Ulcer Advisory Panel (EPUAP) uses a simple, four grade classification. No "ideal" classification system exists; the EPUAP's grade 1 ulceration, for example, may be difficult to detect in people with darkly pigmented skin. Eschar (dried, black, hard, necrotic tissue) covering a pressure ulcer prevents accurate grading. Undermining of adjacent tissue, and sinus wounds, commonly occur and can affect grading as well as healing.

Classification of pressure ulcers by grade*

Grade 1—Non-blanchable erythema of intact skin. Discoloration, warmth, induration, or hardness of skin may also be used as indicators, particularly in people with darker skin

Grade 2—Partial-thickness skin loss, involving epidermis, dermis, or both. The ulcer is superficial and presents clinically as an abrasion or blister

Grade 3—Full-thickness skin loss involving damage to or necrosis of subcutaneous tissue that may extend down to, but not through, underlying fascia

Grade 4—Extensive destruction, tissue necrosis or damage to muscle, bone, or supporting structures, with or without full-thickness skin loss

*As defined by the European Pressure Ulcer Advisory Panel

Prevention and treatment of pressure ulcers

Risk factors

Age alone is not a risk factor; rather, it is the problems common in elderly people that are associated with pressure ulceration. These include hip fractures, faecal and urinary incontinence, smoking, dry skin, chronic systemic conditions, and terminal illness. The effects of all risk factors should be minimised through their optimal management.

Immobility (the inability to reposition without help) and limited activity are probably the major risk factors for pressure ulcers and may occur for various reasons. Elderly people are particularly prone to such problems. Sensory deficits give rise to altered ability to perceive the pain and discomfort associated with persistent local pressure, and this leads to reduced frequency of repositioning.

Being confined to bed or to a chair significantly increases the risk of pressure ulceration; appropriate pressure relieving surfaces should be provided. Individuals with increased limb tone (spasticity) may benefit from interventions such as physiotherapy, muscle relaxants (for example, baclofen), nerve block, or surgery. Care should be taken with the use of sedatives, analgesics, and drugs that cause alteration in skin blood flow, such as antihypertensives.

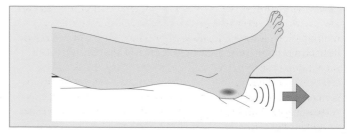

Friction forces generated—for example, when a patient is dragged across a surface

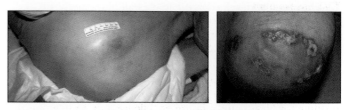

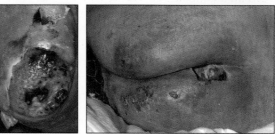

From top left, clockwise: Grade 1 pressure ulcer over greater trochanter; grade 2 pressure ulcers on a below-knee amputation stump due to an ill fitting prosthesis; grade 4 pressure ulcer over the sacrum (with grade 2 pressure ulcers over buttocks); grade 3 pressure ulcer over lateral aspect of calcaneum

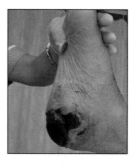

Eschar covering calcaneal pressure ulcer preventing accurate grading

---

Risk factors for pressure ulceration*

Acute illness—Increased metabolic rate and demand for oxygen compromising tissues

Age—Chronic disease, cerebrovascular accident, impaired nutrition, confined to chair or bed, faecal incontinence, fractured neck of femur

Level of consciousness—Acute or chronic illness, medication (sedatives, analgesics, anaesthetics)

Limited mobility or immobility—Cerebrovascular accident, spinal cord injury (hemiparesis, paraparesis, quadriplegia), spasticity, arthritis, orthopaedic problems (especially fracture neck of femur), patients confined to chair or bed

Sensory impairment—Neuropathies (for example, diabetes), decreased conscious levels, medication, spinal cord injury

Severe chronic or terminal disease—Diabetes, chronic obstructive pulmonary disease, chronic cardiovascular disease, terminal illness

Vascular disease—Smoking, diabetes, peripheral vascular disease, anaemia, anti-hypertensives

Malnutrition or dehydration

History of pressure damage

*Based on NICE guidelines for prevention of pressure ulcers

A correlation exists between the degree of malnutrition and the extent and severity of pressure ulceration. In addition, malnutrition slows the healing of pressure ulcers. Measures of nutritional status predictive of pressure ulceration include a recent decrease in body weight, decreased triceps skin-fold thickness, and lymphocytopenia ($< 1.8 \times 10^9$). Serum albumin concentration may be used as a surrogate marker, though its relatively long half life does not provide an accurate reflection of nutritional status. More sensitive markers include serum prealbumin and transferrin concentrations; testing for these, however, is not routinely available.

Risk assessment

A systematic evaluation of risk factors will help to identify patients at risk of pressure ulceration. These individuals should be assessed regularly, and the risk assessment scales should be used as an adjunct to, not a substitute for, clinical judgment. Several risk assessment scales are currently used but vary in the risk factors assessed. The guidelines from the UK National Institute for Health and Clinical Excellence (NICE) state, however, that the provision of pressure relieving devices should also be based on cost considerations and an overall assessment of the individual, not only on risk assessment scores.

NICE recommendations for holistic assessment of patient needing pressure relieving device

- Identified level of risk
- Skin assessment
- Comfort
- General health state
- Lifestyle and abilities
- Critical care needs
- Acceptability of the pressure relieving equipment to patient and carer

---

Pressure relief

Regular inspection of the skin of patients at risk of pressure ulcers should focus particularly on areas around bony prominences. Excess moisture from, for example, urinary or faecal incontinence, perspiration, or wound drainage should be minimised. Patients confined to bed should be turned at least every two hours, the frequency reflecting the type of support surface used and the degree of risk.

Most patients are nursed on a standard hospital mattress. However, those at risk may need to be nursed on a "static" pressure relieving mattress or mattress overlay, which should not be able to "bottom out"—that is, the mattress should not provide less than 2.5 cm of support).

Dynamic mattresses, air-fluidised mattresses, and dynamic overlays provide alternating pressure relief in a cyclical fashion. They are suited to patients at high risk, including those in whom contact of the pressure with the mattress is unavoidable, those with very large or several ulcers, and those with non-healing ulcers.

Direct ("kissing") contact of bony prominences such as the knees and ankles should be avoided by use of cushions or foam wedges. Excess abnormal pressure on the heels should be off-loaded using pressure relieving devices. The patient should not be positioned on the femoral trochanter. Pressure and friction should be minimised by maintaining the head of the bed at less than 30° and using appropriate lifting devices rather than dragging patients during transfer and repositioning.

When sitting in a chair or wheelchair, a patient at risk of pressure ulcers should use a pressure relieving cushion to reduce pressure, ensure good sitting balance, and provide

---

Nutritional support

- Nutritional support is critical in preventing and managing pressure ulcers
- Patients at high risk and those with established ulceration should be assessed and reviewed by a dietitian
- Supplementary feeding, either assisted or enteral (via a nasogastric tube or a percutaneous endoscopic gastrostomy (PEG) tube) may be necessary
- Supplementation with vitamins and trace elements should also be considered
- Adequate hydration is essential

Minimum components of risk assessment scales*

- Age
- Mobility
- Activity
- Level of consciousness
- Nutrition
- Continence
- Skin status
- Illness severity

*Based on NICE recommendations, 2003

Components of three risk assessment scales*

Risk factor	Norton	Waterlow	Braden
Mobility	*Yes*	*Yes*	*Yes*
Activity	Yes	No	Yes
Nutritional status	No	Yes	Yes
Mental status	Yes	No	Yes
Incontinence/moisture	Yes	Yes	Yes
General physical condition	Yes	Yes	No
Skin appearance	No	Yes	No
Medication	No	Yes	No
Friction/shear	No	No	Yes
Weight	No	Yes	No
Age	No	Yes	No
Specific predisposing diseases	No	Yes	No
Prolonged pressure	No	Yes	No

Data from Flanagan M (*J Wound Care* 1993;2:215-8)

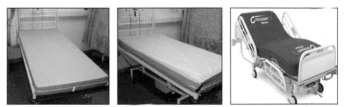

Left to right: Standard hospital mattress; Low tech (Repose) mattress overlay; static mattress

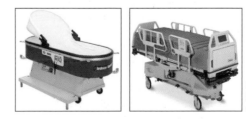

Left: Dynamic mattress. Right: Air-fluidised mattress

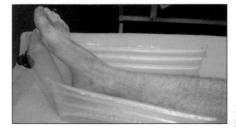

Low tech (Repose) foot protector

comfort. The patient should be encouraged to shift position every 15-30 minutes. If they are unable to do this independently they should be repositioned at least hourly. "Doughnut" or ring cushions should not be used as they may exacerbate rather than prevent the risk of ulceration.

Debridement and dressings

Necrotic or sloughy pressure ulcers should be debrided to promote healing and to enable the stage of the ulcer to be assessed accurately. Devitalised tissue can be removed at the bedside by sharp debridement with a scalpel; local anaesthetic may be needed. Formal surgical debridement may be necessary for extensive grade 3 or 4 pressure ulcers. These ulcers may also require plastic surgery to reconstruct the area. Dressings are the mainstay of treatment of pressure ulcers. Other treatments, including larval and vacuum assisted closure therapies, may be beneficial (see penultimate article in the series).

Complications

All pressure ulcers will be colonised with bacteria. Only signs of clinical infection should prompt bacterial culture to confirm the organism and antibiotic sensitivities. Secondary bacteraemia or septicaemia may complicate pressure ulceration, and each of these conditions is associated with increased mortality. Antibiotics are often started empirically, reflecting the site and depth of the pressure ulcer. A chronic, indolent, non-healing wound may reflect the development of underlying osteomyelitis, the flora of which is often Gram negative or anaerobic (treatment of infection is discussed in a later article). Rarely, amyloidosis or malignancy may arise as a result of chronic pressure ulceration.

The three figures on p 13 and the figure at the top of p 14 are adapted from Grey JE, Harding KG. *Principles and practice of geriatric medicine*. 4th ed. Chichester: Wiley (in press).

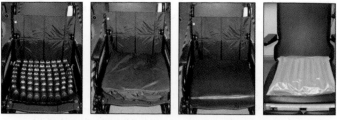

Pressure relieving cushions

Dressing types suitable for the treatment of pressure ulcers pressure ulcer grade

Grade	Dressing type
Grade 1, minimally exuding grade 2	Semipermeable film
Low to moderately exuding, non-infected grades 2-3	Foams
Low to moderately exuding grades 2-4	Hydrogels
Low to moderately exuding grades 3-4	Hydrocolloids
Moderate to highly exuding grades 2-4	Alginates
Moderate to highly exuding grades 2-4	Hydrofibres

Further reading

- European Pressure Ulcer Advisory Panel. *Pressure ulcer prevention guidelines*. www.epuap.org/glprevention.html
- *Pressure relieving devices*. Clinical guidelines. 2003. www.nice.org.uk.
- *Pressure ulcer management*. Clinical guidelines. 2005. www.nice.org.uk
- Cherry GW, Hughes MA, Ferguson MWJ, Leaper DJ. Wound healing. In: Morris DJ, Woods WC, eds. *Oxford textbook of surgery*. 2nd ed. Oxford: Oxford University Press, 2001.
- Clark RAF. *The molecular and cellular biology of wound repair*. 2nd ed. New York: Plenum Press, 1998.
- Glat PM, Longaker MT. Wound healing. In: Aston SJ, Beasley RW, Thorne CHM, eds. *Grabb and Smith's plastic surgery*. 5th ed. Philadelphia, PA: Lippincott- Raven, 1997.
- Brem H, Lyder C. Protocol for the successful treatment of pressure ulcers. *Am J Surg* 2004;188(Suppl 1A):9-17.
- Brem H, Jacobs T, Vileikyte L, Weinberger S, Gibber M, Gill K, et al. Wound-healing protocols for diabetic foot and pressure ulcers. *Surg Technol Int* 2003;11:85-92.
- Cullum N, McInnes E, Bell-Syer SE, Legood R. Support surfaces for pressure ulcer prevention. *Cochrane Database Syst Rev* 2004;(3):CD001735.
- Langer G, Schloemer G, Knerr A, Kuss O, Behrens J. Nutritional interventions for preventing and treating pressure ulcers. *Cochrane Database Syst Rev* 2003;(4):CD003216.

5 Traumatic and surgical wounds

David J Leaper, Keith G Harding

Management of traumatic and surgical wounds has had a chequered history. For example, in 1346 at the Battle of Crécy, France, foot soldiers were issued with cobwebs to staunch haemorrhage caused by trauma. Two centuries later, the eminent surgeon Ambroise Paré (1510-1590) rejected boiling oil as a primary dressing after amputation, preferring a mixture of oil of turpentine, rosewater, and egg.

Classification

Surgical incisions—Surgical incisions cause minimal tissue damage. They are made with precision in an environment where aseptic and antiseptic techniques reduce the risk of infection, with the best of instruments and the facility to control haemostasis. Penetrating trauma may involve minimal damage to skin and connective tissue, though deeper damage to vessels, nerves, and internal organs may occur.

Lacerations—Lacerations are caused when trauma exceeds intrinsic tissue strength—for example, skin torn by blunt injury over a bony prominence such as the scalp. Tissue damage may not be extensive, and primary suturing (see below) may be possible. Sterile skin closure strips may be appropriate in some circumstances—for example, in pretibial laceration, as suturing causes increased tissue tension, with the swelling of early healing and inflammation leading to more tissue loss.

Contusions—Contusions are caused by more extensive tissue trauma after severe blunt or blast trauma. The overlying skin may seem to be intact but later become non-viable. Large haematomas under skin or in muscle may coexist; if they are superficial and fluctuant they can be evacuated with overlying necrosed skin. Ultrasound scanning or magnetic resonance imaging may help to define a haematoma amenable to evacuation. Extensive contusion may lead to infection (antibiotic prophylaxis should be considered in open wounds) and compartment syndromes (fasciotomy will be needed to preserve a limb).

Large open wounds—Such wounds may be left to heal "by secondary intention" (that is, the wound heals from the base upwards, by laying down new tissue) or with delayed skin grafting, depending on the extent of the residual defect. Exploration of a traumatic wound is needed if there is a suspicion of blood vessel or nerve damage, with attention to fractures and debridement of devascularised tissue and removal of foreign material.

Abrasions—Abrasions are superficial epithelial wounds caused by frictional scraping forces. When extensive, they may be associated with fluid loss. Such wounds should be cleansed to minimise the risk of infection, and superficial foreign bodies should be removed (to avoid unsightly "tattooing").

Management

Surgical wounds are made in optimum conditions with full anaesthetic and operating theatre support; traumatic wounds are not, and they may be associated with much more serious underlying injury. Triage and resuscitation may be needed before definitive wound management is started.

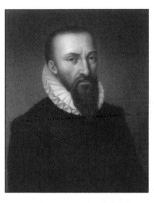

Although the 16th century French surgeon Ambroise Paré could successfully dress a wound, he felt that only God could heal it

Wounds usually involve some loss or damage to an epithelial surface (usually skin) but may also include damage to underlying connective tissue, which may occur without epithelial loss

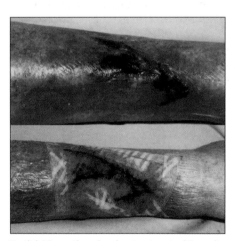

Pretibial laceration showing treatment with sterile skin closure strips

Types of traumatic and surgical wounds

Type of wound	Result	Cause
Incision	*Penetrating*	*Surgical (rarely, trauma)*
Laceration	Torn tissue	Usually trauma
Contusion	Extensive tissue damage	Usually trauma; skin may be intact
Abrasion	Superficial epithelial	Usually trauma
Combination	Usually severe trauma	Life threatening

In England, triage and resuscitation should be done following the Advanced Trauma Life Support guidelines of the Royal College of Surgeons of England (www.rcseng.ac.uk)

ABC of wound healing

Arterial bleeding is easy to recognise—pulsatile and bright red—provided it is overt, but if it is hidden from view (for example, the result of a penetrating injury of the aorta) it may lead to profound unexpected haemorrhagic shock. Early exploration and repair or ligation of blood vessels may be required. Venous haemorrhage is flowing and dark red, and can be controlled by adequate direct pressure. Even large veins may spontaneously stop bleeding after this measure. Capillary bleeding oozes and is bright red; it can lead to shock if injury is extensive and it should not be underestimated.

The risk of infection in traumatic wounds is reduced by adequate wound cleansing and debridement with removal of any non-viable tissue and foreign material. If severe contamination is present, broad spectrum antibiotic prophylaxis is indicated and should be extended as specific therapy as recommended for surgical wounds that are classed as "dirty" or when there are early signs of infection. Traumatic wounds need tetanus prophylaxis (parenteral benzylpenicillin and tetanus toxoid, depending on immune status). Strong evidence supports the use of antibiotic prophylaxis and treatment for surgical wounds that are classed as "clean contaminated" or "contaminated." The value of antibiotic prophylaxis in "clean" wounds is controversial but is widely accepted in prosthetic surgery (such as hip and knee replacement and synthetic vascular bypass surgery).

Wounds from explosions and gunshot

When the source of the wound is high velocity (for example, an explosion or gunshot), it causes more damage because of the dissipation of kinetic energy (kinetic energy $= \frac{1}{2}mv^2$, where m is the mass of the bullet or shrapnel and v its velocity). In addition to gross skeletal injury, soft tissues (such as muscles of the thigh) develop cavitation ahead of the bullet track. These tissues are rendered ischaemic and there may be a large exit wound. Behind the missile there is a sucking action that deposits clothing or dirt in the wound. Together with ischaemia, this contamination provides an ideal culture medium for anaerobic organisms (such as *Clostridium perfringens*, which can lead to gas gangrene).

These wounds need extensive debridement down to viable tissue and should be left open until healthy granulation tissue has formed; repeated debridement may be necessary. Even after extensive debridement, infection may develop, requiring antibiotic treatment. Where there is doubt or an obvious crush injury, fasciotomy can prevent systemic complications, including infection. After debridement, delayed primary or secondary suturing may be done, with or without reconstructive surgery (see eighth article in this series). Alternatively, if the combination of wound contraction and epithelialisation will leave an acceptable cosmetic appearance, a wound may be left to heal by secondary intention. Human and animal bites are traditionally managed in this way, but primary closure can be done after wound debridement and excision of non-viable tissue.

Methods of wound closure

For primary closure, the technique of closure, the suture material, and the type of needle or appliance all need to be considered.

Various suturing techniques exist. Skin may be closed with simple or mattress sutures using interrupted or continuous techniques. Knots should not be tied tightly, to allow swelling as a result of inflammation and to prevent necrosis at the skin edge. Mattress sutures ensure optimal eversion at the skin edge and appose deeper tissue, reducing the risk of formation of haematoma or seroma. The subcuticular suture is the most widely favoured technique for closing surgical skin wounds and

---

> **A tourniquet is rarely needed in traumatic bleeding—control by direct pressure prevents irreversible ischaemia and nerve damage**

Categories of surgical wounds

Category	Example	Recommendation for antibiotics
Clean	Hernia, varicose veins, breast	None
	Prosthetic surgery: vascular, orthopaedic implants	Prophylaxis
Clean contaminated	Elective cholecystectomy	Prophylaxis
Contaminated	Elective colorectal operations	Prophylaxis
Dirty	Drainage of abscess	Treatment if spillage
	Faecal peritonitis	Treatment

> **Bomb blast and gunshot injuries should not be sutured—primarily because of the high risk of infection**

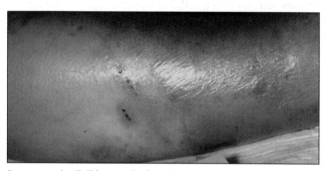

Streptococcal cellulitis complicating a leg wound (wound not shown)

Wounds to consider for open management

- Severe contamination (during laparotomy for faecal peritonitis)
- Old laceration (> 12-24 hours; depends on amount of contusion)
- Shock (of any cause but usually haemorrhagic)
- Devitalisation (local poor tissue perfusion)
- Foreign body (either external or known dead tissue)
- Kinetic energy (in wounds caused by explosions; implies presence of dead tissue and foreign material)

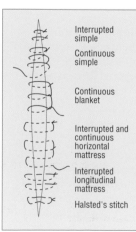

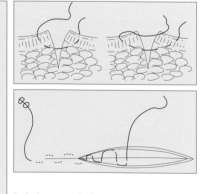

Left: Suture techniques in skin. Top right: Simple and mattress closure. Bottom right: Subcuticular closure

has good cosmetic results. Arterial anastomoses and arteriotomies are closed to ensure eversion, but gut anastomosis conventionally has an inverted suture line.

The ideal suture material for a particular wound remains controversial. Sutures that are absorbable (for example, polyglactin or polydioxanone) clearly do not require removal. Catgut should no longer be used as it causes an excessive tissue reaction, which may predispose to infection. Such reactions are less likely to occur with the use of synthetic polymers. Non-absorbable sutures (for example, natural silk or synthetic polymers such as nylon or polypropylene) need removal. The monofilament polymers cause minimal tissue reaction and are least likely to lead to secondary (exogenous) infection. Silk can cause an intense tissue reaction, with an increased risk of excessive scarring and of formation of a suture abscess; silk is therefore no longer recommended.

Metal clips and staples are alternatives to conventional suturing. Despite their need for removal, they are associated with good cosmetic results and low infection rates. Disposable applicators are expensive but allow rapid closure of long wounds after prolonged surgical procedures. Some stapling devices are sophisticated and allow safer surgery—for example, for very low coloanal anastomosis.

Adhesive strips are useful for closing superficial wounds. In emergency departments a child's forehead laceration can be closed without anaesthetic or tears. They allow for wound swelling and are associated with low infection rates. Adhesive polyurethane film dressings have a similar effect with sutured wounds and provide a barrier to infection. The methacrylate superglues are widely used for skin closure, particularly with scalp wounds (though surrounding hair should be trimmed first). Fibrin glues are relatively expensive but allow rapid closure.

Modern suture materials are presented in sterile, single use packets. Sutures are bonded on to hollow needles. Dispensing with the eye of the needle results in a "shoulderless" needle, permitting easier passage through, and less disruption of, tissues.

Suture removal depends on the wound site. The role of dressings to cover sutured wounds remains controversial. Polyurethane dressings allow inspection and provide a bacterial barrier. Island dressings allow absorbance of wound exudate and lessen the risk of leakage.

Time to removal of non-absorbable sutures

Site of sutures	No of days
Scalp and face	3-4
Upper limb	7
Lower limb	7-10
Trunk	10-14

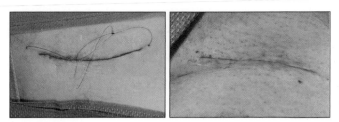

Left: Final appearance of subcuticular closure with polypropylene closure. Right: Final appearance of subcuticular closure with polyglactin closure

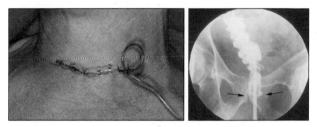

Left: Incision of neck closed with skin clips. Right: X ray showing stapled low anterior resection: the gastrografin enema shows no leakage from the anastomosis

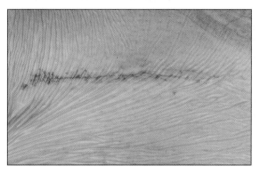

Polyurethane film dressing over a wound after subcuticular closure

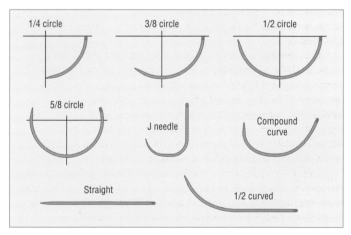

Shapes of needle used in surgical and traumatic wound closure

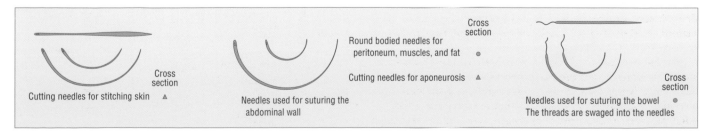

Types of needles used for different surgical procedures. Straight needles and all hand needles are no longer recommended as they have an added risk of causing needle stick injury and the passage of viruses through body fluids. Instrument mounted needles or, when appropriate (as in closure of abdominal fascia), blunted needles should be used

Hidradenitis suppurativa and pilonidal sinus wounds

Hidradenitis, an infection of apocrine sweat glands, affects armpits and groins; pilonidal sinus, a tissue infection caused by in growing hair, mainly affects the natal cleft.

Failed, repeated drainage of the abscesses requires complete excision. The defect usually heals by secondary intention. Initially, excision wounds are usually dressed with polymeric foam. Once the wound has reduced in size, a topical antimicrobial dressing (such as those that contain iodine or silver) may be used. However, grafts or flaps are also used, either as the primary treatment or for non-healing wounds. These wounds often become infected and require prolonged treatment to cover Gram positive and anaerobic organisms.

The picture of Ambroise Paré is published with permission from TopFoto.

Competing interests: DJL has received an educational grant for his research group from Merck Sharp and Dohme and had expenses and a fee paid by Ethicon for attending an advisory panel and for the making of an educational film.

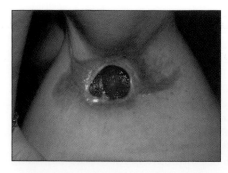

Excision wound in hidradenitis suppurativa

Further reading

- Téot L, Banwell PE, Ziegler UE, eds. *Surgery in wounds*. Berlin: Springer, 2004.
- Leaper DJ, Harding KG, eds. *Wounds. Biology and management*. Oxford: Oxford Medical Publications, 1998.
- Bales S, Harding K, Leaper DJ. *An introduction to wounds*. London: Emap Healthcare, 2000.
- Leaper DJ, Harding KG, Phillips CJ. Management of wounds. In: Johnson C, Taylor I, eds. *Recent advances in surgery*. 25th ed. London: Royal Society of Medicine, 2002.
- Leaper DJ, Low L. Surgical access: incisions and the management of wounds. In: Kirk RM, Ribbons WJ, eds. *Clinical surgery in general*. 4th ed. Edinburgh: Churchill Livingstone, 2004.
- Leaper DJ. Basic surgical skills and anastomoses. In: Russell RCG, Williams NS, Bulstrode CJK, eds. *Bailey and Love's short practice of surgery*. 24th ed. London: Arnold, 2004.

6 Uncommon causes of ulceration

Girish K Patel, Joseph E Grey, Keith G Harding

This chapter describes some of the many rare causes of ulceration. Rare causes that are more common in developing countries—such as leprosy, fungal infections, Buruli ulcer, and ulceration resulting from Kaposi sarcoma—are not covered here.

Inflammatory disorders

Inflammatory disorders can lead to ulceration or impair healing directly or through the effect of medication used to treat the disorder; ulceration is a feature of many connective tissue diseases. For example, ulceration develops in up to 10% of patients with rheumatoid arthritis and is often painful. In addition to the underlying disease, impaired healing can result from anaemia, skin atrophy, dependent oedema, deformity, neuropathy, microvascular disease, local factors, or the toxic effects of drugs used in its treatment. Other associated conditions such as vasculitis or pyoderma gangrenosum may also lead to ulceration.

Ulceration in rheumatoid arthritis is usually of rapid onset or enlargement, associated with pain (not relieved by raising or lowering the leg), fever, malaise, arthralgia, and myalgia. The ulcer may be multifocal and/or have an atypical location, tender margin, and/or a violaceous or erythematous inflammatory border.

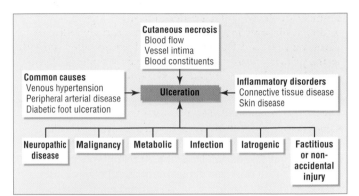

Causes of ulceration, according to typical clinical presentation

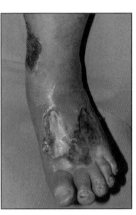

Rheumatoid arthritis on dorsum of foot with exposed tendon, and over medial malleolus; such ulcers have a smooth, irregular margin

---

Connective tissue disease associated with ulceration

- Rheumatoid arthritis
- Systemic lupus erythematosus
- Dermatomyositis
- Systemic sclerosis
- Sjögren's syndrome
- Behçet's syndrome

Treatment of ulceration related to connective tissue disease may require immunosuppressants, including steroids and/or cytotoxic agents

Pyoderma gangrenosum

Pyoderma gangrenosum is characterised by the appearance of lesions at the site of trauma (for example, venepuncture). Surgical debridement of pyoderma gangrenosum often leads to a worsening of the ulceration. The diagnosis of pyoderma gangrenosum is primarily clinical but may be associated with specific features on histology. The patient often has a history of a painful sterile pustule or nodule with surrounding erythema, which eventually ruptures and ulcerates. The ulcer has a characteristic erythematous or violaceous overhanging edge. The wound bed is often purulent and may extend to muscle. Over half of cases of pyoderma gangrenosum are associated with underlying active or quiescent systemic disease; these include inflammatory bowel disease, seronegative rheumatoid arthritis, and lymphoproliferative diseases. Treatment of pyoderma gangrenosum is usually with immunosuppressants.

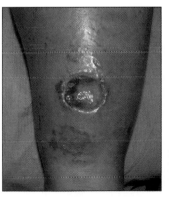

Pyoderma gangrenosum over posterior gaiter area of leg (note also allergy to dressing on surrounding skin)

Necrobiosis lipoidica

Necrobiosis lipoidica commonly presents as a pretibial yellowish atrophic plaque. It is often associated with diabetes mellitus and has a propensity to ulcerate, usually as a result of minor trauma. Typically, such ulceration is slow to heal, painful, and often complicated by infection. In most cases the ulceration

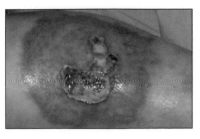

Necrobiosis lipoidica complicated by ulceration in centre

will heal with good wound care and the use of potent topical corticosteroids to the surrounding lesion.

Skin necrosis

Skin necrosis is a manifestation of tissue death that occurs as a consequence of rapid ischaemia, often due to vessel occlusion. The pattern and extent of necrosis varies according to the size of the vessels affected. In the 1860s, Rudolf Virchow proposed that thrombus formation is attributable to a change in three components: blood flow, the vessel intima, and blood constituents. This proposal (Virchow's triad) provides a useful framework to consider the causes of skin necrosis.

Blood flow

Rapid reduction in local blood flow that may arise from an embolic event, severe chilblains, and Raynaud's phenomenon can present with dramatic digital necrosis. All patients with Raynaud's phenomenon should be advised not to smoke cigarettes and to reduce caffeine intake. Both primary and secondary Raynaud's phenomenon may respond well to conservative measures, including cold avoidance and treatment with a long acting calcium channel antagonist or another oral vasodilator. Topical vasodilators—for example, glyceryl trinitrate—may also be of benefit. In severe chronic disease, cervical sympathectomy can be done; in severe acute necrotising disease, infusions with prostaglandin E1 or epoprostenol (prostacyclin) can save digits.

Vessel intima

Calciphylaxis is characterised by painful, haemorrhagic skin necrosis with a reticulate edge. Skin histology shows vessel intramural hyperplasia, intravascular calcification, and thrombosis. Calciphylaxis most often occurs in patients with renal failure who are having dialysis or patients with hyperparathyroidism, or idiopathically. Treatment consists of analgesia, removal of calcium deposits at the site of any ulceration, and control of predisposing factors.

Almost all types of vasculitis can present with skin necrosis. In some cases, such as Wegener's granulomatosis and classic polyarteritis nodosa, they can be a cause of chronic ulceration. Vasculitis is classified according to the size of vessel affected. Medium sized vessel vasculitis presents with painful nodules that may ulcerate. Small vessel vasculitis typically presents with palpable purpura.

Blood constituents

Several coagulation factors are associated with skin necrosis and are due either to genetic or acquired alteration in function. Some syndromes are also associated with hypercoagulability.

Antiphospholipid syndrome is a heterogeneous group of disorders characterised by the presence of autoantibodies against various phospholipids, including lupus anticoagulant and anticardiolipin. The disorder affects mostly females and may be associated with systemic lupus erythematosus. Antiphospholipid syndrome may present as a cause of multiple arterial and venous thrombotic episodes, recurrent spontaneous abortions, and the presence of livedo reticularis. Antiphospholipid syndrome is a cause of livedoid vasculopathy, a disorder characterised by painful ulceration in association with livedo reticularis and atrophie blanche. Livedoid vasculopathy has also been described as being associated with factor V Leiden mutation. This progressive, painful, and debilitating disease requires anticoagulation, plus drugs to treat the underlying disease.

> **Topical PUVA (psoralens and ultraviolet A) therapy may also have a role in necrobiosis lipoidica**

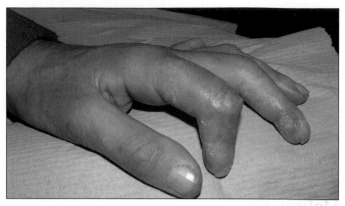

Ulcerations due to Raynaud's phenomenon over proximal interphalangeal joint of index finger (associated with infection) and over distal interphalangeal joint of middle finger

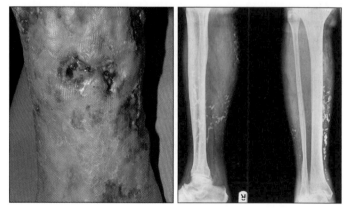

Left: Calciphylaxis showing calcium deposits in base of ulcer. Right: X ray of same patient showing extensive subcutaneous calcification

Causes of vasculitis, classified according to size of vessel affected*

Large vessel	Medium vessel	Small vessel
Giant cell (temporal) arteritis	*Classic polyarteritis nodosa*	*Wegener's granulomatosis; Churg-Strauss syndrome; microscopic polyangiitis*
Takayasu's arteritis	Kawasaki disease	Henoch-Schönlein purpura; essential cryoglobulinaemic vasculitis; cutaneous leukocytoclastic angiitis

*Chapel Hill consensus conference, 1992.

Abnormalities of coagulation factors associated with skin necrosis

- Protein C deficiency
- Protein S deficiency
- Antithrombin 3 deficiency
- Heparin cofactor 2 deficiency
- Homocystinaemia
- Raised prothrombin concentrations
- Factor 12 deficiency
- Factor V Leiden mutation

Warfarin necrosis is an uncommon transient phenomenon, which occurs at the start of warfarin treatment in the absence of heparin. The condition affects mostly females, and individuals are usually in their 50s or 60s. It typically involves sites abundant in subcutaneous fat, such as breasts, hip, buttock, and thigh. The use of warfarin results in a transient decrease of vitamin K sensitive factors, including protein C, resulting in a temporary hypercoagulable state, which spontaneously corrects itself. Warfarin should therefore be continued.

Heparin necrosis is rare and may be caused by both unfractionated and low molecular weight heparin. It is associated with the formation of antibodies, leading to platelet clumping. The continued use of heparin leads to greater platelet clumping and emboli affecting both cutaneous and internal organs. Skin necrosis occurs at injection and distant sites. Heparin aggravates the condition, with potentially fatal consequences, so it should be stopped immediately.

Malignancy

Many types of cancers, including metastases, present with skin ulceration, including the commonest forms of skin cancer, basal cell carcinoma, and squamous cell carcinoma. Although the incidence of squamous cell carcinoma increases with age, it may present in younger individuals with a genetic predisposition or with a history of excessive exposure to ultraviolet light, of organ transplantation, or of immunosuppressants (such as ciclosporin).

Squamous cell carcinoma may also develop in longstanding chronic ulceration associated with burns, scalds, radiotherapy, or venous disease (Marjolin's ulcer). Features indicative of malignancy include rapid enlargement of the lesion despite conventional treatment; pain; bleeding; and often a rolled edge. Squamous cell carcinoma arising in longstanding chronic ulcers can exhibit a more aggressive phenotype, with a greater potential to metastasise. In most cases of lower leg skin cancer the preferred treatment is surgical excision. However, in cases of substantial comorbidity or disseminated metastatic disease, palliative treatment (radiotherapy and local wound care) may be more appropriate.

Drug and iatrogenic causes

Hydroxycarbamide (hydroxyurea), used to treat myeloproliferative diseases, may cause a painful, shallow, lower leg ulcer, usually over the medial malleolus, up to 15 years after start of treatment. Healing is normally only achieved when hydroxycarbamide is discontinued.

Radiotherapy, used to treat benign and malignant diseases, is associated with an endarteritis that may result in ulceration and impair wound healing. Furthermore, after radiotherapy the skin is at risk of ulceration as a result of chronic radiation dermatitis, allergic contact dermatitis, squamous cell carcinoma, and angiosarcoma.

Factitious

Factitious wounds and non-accidental injury can also present as atypical wounds. Often the patient's history is incongruent with the clinical appearance of the wound. Further clues can be gained from the pattern of the lesion and from a skin biopsy (useful for excluding disease and for identifying the presence of foreign material). Occasionally, admission to hospital is necessary to verify the diagnosis. The management of such cases invariably relies on a multidisciplinary approach involving a liaison psychiatrist.

> ***Purpura fulminans*** **includes three different syndromes (neonatal; associated with sepsis; and postinfective) associated with widespread capillary and venule thrombosis that present as purpura and skin necrosis. Skin necrosis favours the extremities, particularly the digits. *Purpura fulminans* is a complication of either hereditary or acquired protein C or protein S deficiency**

Infection

- β-haemolytic *Streptococcus pyogenes* and *Staphylococcus aureus* are responsible for many of the infections that can complicate existing ulceration
- They may also in certain circumstances be the cause of ulceration. β-haemolytic streptococcus may lead to erysipelas, bullous cellulitis, punched out ulceration (ecthyma) and necrotising fasciitis
- When the patient has a history of foreign travel, then *Leishmania*, atypical mycobacterium, and deep mycotic infection should also be considered as causes of ulceration
- In patients with AIDS or other immunosuppressive states, ulceration may indicate infection with syphilis, tuberculosis, bacillary angiomatosis, herpes simplex, or cytomegalovirus infection

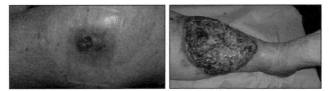

Left: Basal cell carcinoma presenting over medial aspect of knee; note evidence of biopsy of centre of lesion and orange coloration (due to dressing containing iodine). Right: Florid, ulcerating, necrotic squamous cell carcinoma of lower leg

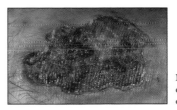

Marjolin's ulcer—a squamous cell carcinoma arising as a complication of longstanding venous leg ulceration

Further reading
- Enoch S, Kupitz S, Miller DR, Harding KG. Dystrophic calcification as a cause for non-healing leg ulcers. *Int Wound J* 2005;2:142-7.
- Enoch S, Miller DR, Harding KG, Price PE. Early diagnosis is vital in the management of squamous cell carcinomas associated with chronic non-healing ulcers: a case series and review of the literature. *Int Wound J* 2004;1:165-75.
- Rovee DT, Maibach HI. *The epidermis in wound healing*. Boca Raton, Fl: CRC Press, 2003.
- Falanga V, ed. *Cutaneous wound healing*. London: Martin Dunitz, 2001.
- Leaper DJ, Harding KG, eds. *Wound: biology and management*. Oxford: Oxford Medical, 1998.

7 Burns

Alex Benson, William A Dickson, Dean E Boyce

About 250 000 people are burnt each year in the United Kingdom. Of these, almost 112 000 attend an accident and emergency department and about 210 die of their injuries. At least 250 000 others attend their general practitioner for treatment of their injury. A burn results in loss of epidermal integrity of the skin; this article discusses the aetiology and management of various types of burn injury.

Mechanisms of burn

Thermal injury

Flame—Accelerants such as petrol, lighter fluid, or natural gas are often involved. The depth of flame burn is typically full or partial thickness.

Scald—60% of burns in children are from scalds. Non-accidental injury is rare but should be considered if there are delays in presentation, inconsistencies in history, or an unusual pattern of injury.

Contact—Contact burns often present as small burns on extremities, but they can be serious in those not able to remove themselves from the source of injury, such as elderly people, children, disabled people, and those incapacitated by drugs, alcohol, fit, or faint.

Flash—Flash burns are usually to the face and upper limbs and are caused by an explosive ignition of a volatile substance. They are often due to use of accelerants to light a fire or gas explosions.

Electrical injury

Low voltage—The energy imparted from 240 V usually gives a deep burn in the form of a small entry and exit wound. Such burns are commonly seen on the hands. If alternating current crosses the myocardium, arrhythmias may arise. If the electrocardiogram is normal and there is no history of loss of consciousness, admission to hospital for cardiac monitoring is not required.

High voltage—High tension burns occur with an injury resulting from 1000 V or more. These catastrophic injuries result in extensive tissue damage. Rhabdomyolysis and renal failure may occur.

Flash—An arc of high tension current from a high voltage power source may cause injury, without the current traversing the body. Heat can damage exposed skin, and clothing may ignite.

Chemical injury

Acids—Acids cause coagulative necrosis, denature proteins, and are usually painful. Hydrofluoric acid penetrates tissues deeply and can cause fatal systemic toxicity even in small burns. Immediate copious lavage and treatment with topical calcium gluconate gel is essential. Systemic calcium may be required as hydrofluoric acid sequesters calcium with the burn.

Alkalis—Common household alkalis such as bleaches, cleaning agents, and cement give a liquefactive necrosis. They have the potential to penetrate tissues deeper than most acids as further injury occurs as cells dehydrate and collagen and protein are denatured. Often the onset of pain is delayed, thus postponing first aid and allowing more tissue damage.

Aetiology of burn injuries (percentage)

Adults	Paediatric
● Flame (48)	● Scalds (60)
● Scalds* (33)	● Flame (25)
● Contact (8)	● Contact (10)
● Electrical (5)	● Electrical (2)
● Chemical (3)	● Chemical (2)
● Friction (2)	● Sunburn (1)
● Sunburn (1)	

Adapted from UK manual for "Emergency Management of Severe Burns" course. See also next page
*Oil and water.

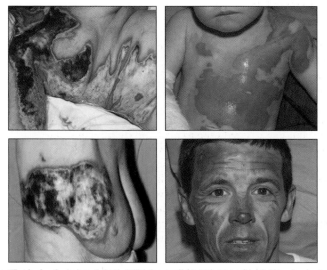

Clockwise from top left: Full thickness flame burn to the right arm, torso, and face and neck (not shown); "pull over" scald (hot tea) to a toddler; flash burn and erythema to face (note sparing of skin creases); full thickness contact burn (patient was alcoholic and fell unconscious against a portable heater)

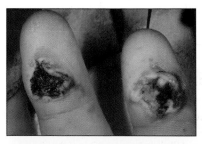

Low voltage (240 V) electrical burns to the finger pulps

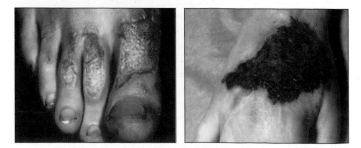

Left: Cement burns to the dorsum of the toe. These burns may initially be deemed superficial; persistence of the alkali within the skin can cause a progressive full thickness burn. Right: Full thickness caustic soda burn

Burn assessment

The severity of burn injuries is related to the depth of skin involvement and the percentage of total body surface area involved.

In the United Kingdom burns are classified as partial thickness or full thickness, as these terms correspond to the level of burn injury and the likelihood of healing without surgical intervention.

Partial thickness burns are further categorised as superficial or deep dermal. Superficial burns usually heal without surgery, but deeper burns are likely to require excision and skin grafts. Burn depth can progress without adequate first aid and treatment such as appropriate fluid resuscitation and dressings. Burn depth can be worsened by the presence of infection. Superadded infection may lead to an increase in burn depth.

Classification of burn depth

Superficial burns

These usually heal within 14 days and leave minimal scarring. Burn erythema may be described as skin redness and pain. Erythema is not included in the assessment of the percentage of total body surface area. With superficial dermal burns the outer part of the dermis is injured; these burns characteristically have blisters and are very painful.

Deep burns

These take a prolonged time to heal and do so with severe scarring. All but the smallest areas of full thickness burn require surgical intervention. In deep dermal burns the skin has fixed capillary staining and has blotchy cherry red appearance. It does not blanch with pressure and is typically insensate. Full thickness burns have a leathery white or charred black appearance (eschar). In people with dark skin, parameters other than skin colour may need to be used.

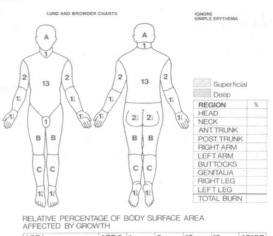

A Lund and Browder chart is useful in assessing the extent of burn injury (the relative proportions of body areas differ in children)

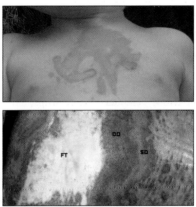

Top: Superficial dermal scald (top). Bottom: Burn injury of different depths (FT= full thickness; DD = deep dermal; SD = superficial dermal)

Indicators of depth of burn injury

Burn type	Skin colour	Blisters	Capillary refill	Sensation	Pinprick	Healing
Epidermal	Red	Absent	Brisk	Painful	Bleeds	Yes
Superficial dermal	Pale pink	Present (small)	Brisk	Painful	Bleeds	Yes
Mid-dermal	Dark pink	Present	Slow	May be painful	Bleeds	Usually
Deep dermal	Dry blotchy red	May be present	Absent	No pain	No bleeding	No
Full thickness	Dry white/black	Absent	Absent	No pain	No bleeding	No

Management of burn injuries

First aid

The person should be removed from the burning source without endangering the rescuers. If clothing is alight, follow the "drop and roll" procedure. When electricity is involved, power should be turned off before administering first aid.

The burn should be cooled (or the toxin diluted) with lukewarm running water for at least 20 minutes. This period should be increased in those with chemical injury. Ice or very cold water should be avoided, as blood flow to the affected area will be reduced, and hypothermia induced, particularly in infants and elderly people.

Patients are assessed and their treatment priorities established on the basis of the severity of their injuries The history of events leading to the burn will also alert those treating the patient to the risks of coexisting injury. Inhalation injury is potentially life threatening when burns have been sustained in enclosed areas.

The "drop and roll" procedure: get the person to drop to the ground then help them to roll over to extinguish the flames from burning clothing (the use of a wet blanket may help)

Protocol for managing burn injuries*

A = Airway and cervical spine control
B = Breathing and ventilation
C = Circulation and haemorrhage control
D = Disability
E = Exposure and environmental control
F = Fluid resuscitation

*According to guidelines advocated in the course "Emergency Management of Severe Burns," run by the British Burn Association (www.britishburnsassociation.co.uk)

Simple analgesia or opiates should be used. Covering the burn and cooling with water will also provide some pain relief.

Dressings

Polyvinyl chloride sheeting ("clingfilm") or sterile cotton sheeting may be used initially. These are simple to use and allow wound inspection so that definitive assessment can be performed. Sterile burn cooling gels are also available.

Minor burn injury

Debridement

Burn debris should be removed with mild soap and water, sterile saline, or a topical antiseptic solution before dressings are applied. The dead skin of open blisters should be removed, and large or friable blisters should also be "deroofed" (the outer layer removed). Small blisters may be left intact. Antibiotics are not routinely prescribed in minor burns. The tetanus status of the patient should be checked.

Dressings

In the simple, clean, partial thickness burn, dressings such as paraffin gauze (for example, Jelonet), chlorhexidine impregnated gauze (Bactigras), or similar dressings such as soft silicone (Mepitel) or soft polymer (Urgotul) can be used with an overlying gauze pad. Hydrocolloid dressings are particularly good for use on hands and other small areas of superficial or partial thickness burns, although they leave a "skim" of exudate that needs to be removed to allow appropriate assessment of the wound. In bigger burns, several layers of dressing are usually required to absorb exudate and to prevent shear or friction of the skin.

Dressings such as alginate adhere to the wound and should be reviewed after 24 hours. At this point only the secondary dressing immediately overlying the alginate needs to be replaced. Once the wound is healed, the alginate separates off. If there is excessive exudate or a full thickness burn, the dressing fails to stick, indicating the necessity for further assessment. These properties also make alginate dressings useful for donor sites after skin graft harvest.

Major burn injury

A major burn should be managed according to the guidelines advocated in the British Burn Association's Emergency Management of Severe Burns course. Transfer of these patients needs careful planning and communication with the burns team. In a patient with multiple injuries, the most obvious injury may be their burn, but careful assessment and treatment of other injuries is vital before burn management. All patients with facial burns or suspected of having inhaled smoke or hot gases should be assessed by an anaesthetist before being transferred to a specialist unit , as early intubation may be required.

Deep or full thickness burns make the skin inelastic and act like a tourniquet. They should be released by escharotomy to prevent respiratory embarrassment (of the chest and abdomen) or vascular compromise of the limbs. This may need to be done before transfer to a specialist unit.

Fluid resuscitation is indicated after a serious burn ($\geq 10\%$ of total body surface area in children and $\geq 15\%$ in adults). The British Burn Association recommends the use of the Parkland formula, but intravenous fluids should also be guided by the patient's response to resuscitation.

Surgical debridement of the major burn is influenced by the fitness of the patient to undergo a procedure and the depth and location of the burn. Excision of the burn may be required. Reconstruction is often done with split skin grafts taken from the patient in single or multiple stages. This may be combined

> All burns are susceptible to infection. Silver based products have traditionally been used to treat burns, including silver sulfadiazine (Flamazine) and silver sulfadiazine plus cerous nitrate (Flammacerium)—the latter available only on a named patient basis in the UK. However, the use of these preparations makes subsequent assessment difficult. Ideally, they should not be applied without discussion with the burns team

Criteria for referral to a burns centre

- Associated airway injury
- Partial thickness burns >5% of total body surface area in a child
- Partial thickness burns >10% of total body surface area in an adult
- >1% full thickness burn
- Partial or full thickness burns to face, perineum, external genitalia, feet and hands, and over joints
- Circumferential injury
- Chemical and electrical burns
- Extremes of age
- Non-accidental injury
- Comorbidity
- Non-healed burn three weeks after injury

> Repeated review of the burn wound and multiple dressing changes are unnecessary. A change of dressings and wound review after 48 hours is usual. Further changes are guided by the rate of healing, but are generally needed at intervals of two to three days. More frequent change of dressing is needed if there is a high volume of exudate or evidence of infection

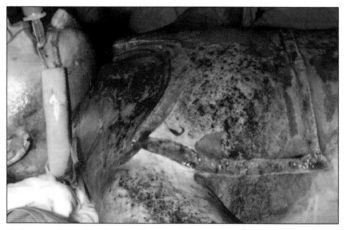

Escharotomies to the chest to allow respiratory expansion

Fluid resuscitation guide based on Parkland formula

Calculations are guidelines only and refer to fluid required from the time of burn injury, not the time of presentation. Volumes refer to fluid resuscitation for the first 24 hours: half is given in the first 8 hours, and half over the subsequent 16 hours

Resuscitation formula for adults
- 3-4 ml Hartmann's solution/kg body weight/% total body surface area

Resuscitation formula for children
- 3-4 ml Hartmann's solution/kg body weight/% total body surface area, plus maintenance fluids (4% glucose in 0.25N saline or 0.2N saline)

with cadaveric skin if the patient has insufficient donor skin. Artificial skin substitutes are being increasingly used with good results (see a later article in this series). Several layers of dressings are used to minimise shear at the site of skin grafting. These should not be too tight as swelling often occurs after a burn injury.

Once a burn has healed, the area should be regularly moisturised and protected from the sun by sunblock cream or clothing. Physiotherapy may be required to prevent burn contractures.

Further reading and resources

- Herndon D. *Total burn care*. 2nd ed. London: Saunders, 2002.
- National Burn Care Review. National burn injury referral guidelines. In: *Standards and strategy for burn care*. London: NBCR, 2001:68-9.
- Burnsurgery.org (a website designed to be a comprehensive educational tool for burn care professionals worldwide) www.burnsurgery.org

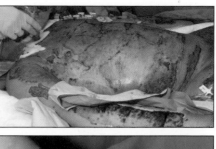

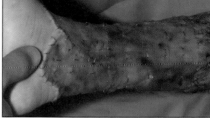

Top: Full thickness burns of the abdomen have been excised and closed with split thickness skin grafts. Bottom: Artificial skin substitute used to cover full thickness burn

Prevention of burns is key: the main improvement in reduction of burns in the UK over the past 40 years has been the introduction of legislation to reduce the flammability of clothing, furniture, and fireworks and of proper labelling of inflammable materials

8 Reconstructive surgery

Dean E Boyce, Kayvan Shokrollahi

Many surgical options are available to a reconstructive surgeon when faced with a difficult wound. However, any decision about management should be holistic and take into account factors such as the occupational circumstances of the patient and likely period of time off work, comorbidity, likelihood of success, donor morbidity, functional outcome, and the risks of surgery and anaesthesia. The basic principles of wound management apply to all wounds.

The "reconstructive ladder"

Reconstructive surgeons use the concept of a "reconstructive ladder"—the more problematic the wound, the higher up the ladder the surgeon has to climb. Simple wounds may be closed by primary suturing, sometimes in the primary care setting. But others may require complex reconstruction, including free tissue transfer, in hospital.

All traumatic wounds should undergo debridement and thorough irrigation before primary closure. The aim of debridement is to remove all potentially contaminated and devitalised tissue along with foreign material. Primary suture may not be indicated in heavily contaminated wounds, where the risk of infection is high. In such cases the wound should be debrided, with "delayed closure" carried out later. Occasionally, wounds may be allowed to heal by secondary intention, where areas of skin loss are initially replaced by granulation tissue. The skin defect continues to heal as a result of proliferation or migration of epidermal cells within and around the wound and by contraction of the wound by specialised cells (myofibroblasts) within the granulation tissue. Healing by secondary intention is slow and may lead to contractures, scarring, and restriction of movements.

Where skin defects are too large for skin apposition, and healing by secondary intention is inappropriate, skin grafts may be used. Free skin grafts are taken from another part of the body and rely on revascularisation from a healthy, well vascularised wound bed. Grafts will not be successful on non-vascularised beds, such as exposed bone or tendon.

Split skin grafts consist of the epidermis and a variable amount of dermis. They are usually harvested from the thigh using a specially designed knife or powered dermatome. The donor area will heal within 10-14 days from remaining dermal adnexal structures. Such grafts are the mainstay of treatment of large wounds such as burns. Full thickness grafts consist of the epidermis and dermis and offer several advantages, but are size limited as the donor area must be directly closed.

Expansion of local skin using subcutaneous tissue expanders is a method of increasing the amount of skin locally available. A tissue expander is placed beneath the skin and inflated at weekly intervals by injecting saline through a remote port. The overlying tissue expands in response to mechanical force. Epidermal thickness increases as a result of cellular hyperplasia. The dermis also undergoes increased fibroplasia, with realignment of collagen fibres and disruption of elastic fibres. This also results, however, in a reduction in dermal thickness and separation of dermal appendages, such as hair follicles.

The surgical management of problem wounds generally aims to obtain rapid wound closure with the simplest method and with minimal compromise of cosmesis and function

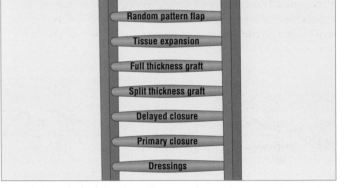

Free flap
Pedicled flap
Random pattern flap
Tissue expansion
Full thickness graft
Split thickness graft
Delayed closure
Primary closure
Dressings

The "reconstructive ladder" is used by reconstructive surgeons to assess the complexity of treatment required

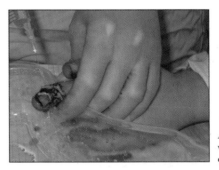

A finger injury is irrigated with saline before debridement and closure

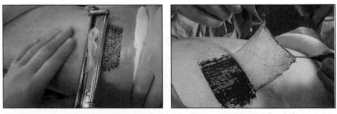

Harvesting a split thickness skin graft using a hand held knife

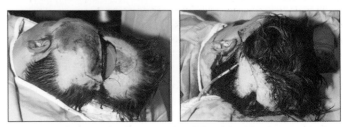

A tissue expander has been used to expand the right side of the scalp to reconstruct the wound left after excision of a congenital melanocyic naevus

Many wounds, such as fracture sites and exposed bone or tendon, are not suitable for grafting, and techniques further up the reconstructive ladder, such as a flap reconstruction, must be used. A flap is a unit of tissue that can be moved to cover a wound while surviving on its own vascular supply. Random pattern flaps rely on random cutaneous vessels for their blood supply.

Greater lengths of flap can be used by including the underlying deep fascia and also by including a perforating blood vessel in the base of the flap. In some circumstances better cosmesis may be obtained by raising the flap as fascia only, leaving the overlying skin behind. "Islanding" a flap on its vascular pedicle allows even greater pedicle length and thus greater mobility and versatility. Occasionally no options are available for local wound cover, and tissue has to be harvested from elsewhere around the body by using microvascular techniques. This transfer of tissue, known as a free flap, represents the top rung of the reconstructive ladder. Any tissue that can be isolated on a suitable vascular pedicle can be used, and it may include muscle, skin, fascia, fat, nerve, and bone.

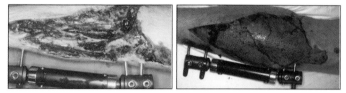

Left: Compound tibial fracture. Right: Wound closure of the fracture using a free latissimus dorsi muscle flap covered with a split thickness skin graft

Specific wounds

Pressure ulcers
When considering surgery for pressure ulcers, bear in mind that the wound will recur if the original precipitant is still present. Surgical intervention may sometimes be required, once intrinsic and extrinsic factors have been resolved. Some units have "outreach" pressure ulcer teams who will give treatment and advice both in the community and on the wards. Surgery should be a last resort and would consist of an "oncological" debridement of the ulcer (including any areas of osteomyelitis) and excision of bony prominences. Direct closure is usually not possible, and a local closure using a fasciocutaneous or myocutaneous flap is usually necessary.

Necrotising infections
Acute infections such as necrotising fasciitis can cause rapid tissue loss in a very short time. They have polymicrobial aetiology, and the classic Lancefield group A β haemolytic streptococci may be present in only 15% of cases. After adequate resuscitation, appropriate antibiotics and prompt surgical debridement of affected areas may be life saving, and the patient would need a period of intensive support. Significant tissue destruction can occur in minutes, highlighting the importance of rapid debridement, and subsequently large body surface areas may require surgical reconstruction, most often with split skin grafts. Flap coverage may occasionally be needed when the bed is not suitable for a graft.

Arterial ulcers
Peripheral vascular disease can be a primary cause of ulceration and poor wound healing and is often a contributory reason for poor healing of wounds from other causes. Bypass grafting or angioplasty to improve arterial input to the distal limb can be curative in itself or can be done to enable other forms of

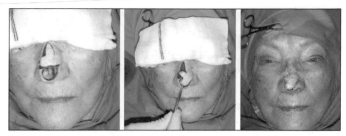

Left to right: Excision of a tumour has left a defect on the nasal tip (the flaps have been raised but not transposed); the flap is transposed into the defect, and the adjacent flap is transposed into the donor area; final result. This procedure is an example of a random patterned flap

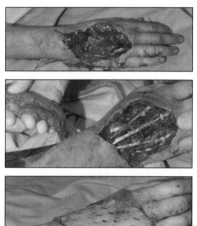

Top: Defect on the back of the hand showing exposed fractures and destroyed tendons (this is unsuitable for skin grafting). Centre: At reconstruction a distally based adipofascial flap has been raised using the radial artery as a pedicle; the overlying donor skin is closed primarily. Bottom: The flap is inset and covered by a split skin graft

> **Most wound types outlined in this section are discussed in more detail in previous articles in this series**

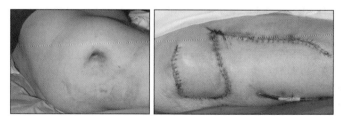

Left: Chronic trochanteric pressure ulcer excised. Right: Reconstruction using a tensor fascia lata myocutaneous flap

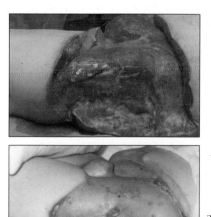

Top: Necrotising fasciitis of the groin after surgical debridement. Bottom: Wound closure with a split thickness skin graft

reconstruction that otherwise would fail (such as grafts or flaps). Other indications for surgery include the debridement of necrotic or infected tissue. In circumstances of chronic non-healing, sepsis, or long term disability, amputation of digits or limbs is often the best solution to enable rapid healing and improve quality of life. With appropriate counselling from the multidisciplinary team (surgeon, prosthetist, specialist nurses, physiotherapist, occupational therapist, and general practitioner), patients can make informed decisions about such treatments. Prosthetists can advise the surgeon on the level of amputation required taking into account the most up to date or suitable artificial aids.

Diabetic foot ulcers

After proximal arterial disease has been excluded, hypertrophic keratinous edges of ulcers are debrided and pressure points "off loaded" (relieved of pressure) by use of appropriate orthoses, although bony prominences and areas of osteomyelitis may need to be excised. If, despite adequate treatment and graft or flap closure, ulceration and infection recurs, amputation may be the best treatment.

Pilonidal sinus and abscess

Chronic sinuses are excised down to the sacral fascia. The wound is allowed to heal by secondary intention or closed with the aid of "Z plasty" (a procedure involving transposition of two interdigitating triangular flaps that elongate and change direction of the common limb of the flap) or a local flap.

Non-melanoma skin cancer

Basal cell carcinoma and squamous cell carcinoma are the two commonest types of skin cancer and are often characterised by ulceration. In addition, squamous cell carcinoma can develop in any chronic wound. Treatment of these lesions requires excision with a suitable margin (typically 3 mm for basal cell and 5 mm for squamous cell carcinoma). Preoperative microbiology testing and perioperative antibiotics are recommended for excision of ulcerated lesions, as such excisions are associated with increased rates of surgical wound infection. Radiotherapy, curettage, cryosurgery, and photodynamic therapy—as well as a number of new topical treatments—may be used in the treatment of basal cell carcinoma, but none of these procedures can provide definitive histology or match adequate surgery in terms of recurrence rates.

Hidradenitis suppurativa

Surgery entails excision of the affected area, leaving a large skin wound. Primary closure of the wound is usually not possible. Healing by secondary intention involves many weeks of dressings and a substantial risk of scar contracture. Skin grafts may be used, but these run the risk of resulting in scar contracture and delayed healing. Flap reconstruction may result in more rapid wound closure and a reduced risk of contracture.

The authors thank R Kannan, M S C Murison, D S Murray, T Potokar, G D Sterne, and O G Titley for help in providing clinical photographs.

Venous leg ulcers

- Surgery, if indicated, may include application of split skin graft onto a healthy ulcer bed, pinch grafting (several small islands of epidermis from a healthy donor site applied to the wound bed), and excision of the ulcer and treatment with split skin grafts
- These techniques may enable more rapid healing than dressings and compression alone. However, this is at the cost of a donor site wound, which may be slow to heal because of infection or other comorbidities, such as diabetes
- More complex procedures, such as coverage with a flap, may be required if tendon or bone is exposed. Tissue engineered skin substitutes have been used (see 12th article in this series), but this technique remains an expensive and unconventional treatment

> **With a diabetic foot ulcer, amputation may be in the form of a ray amputation, or an amputation at the level of forefoot, midfoot, hind foot, or below the knee**

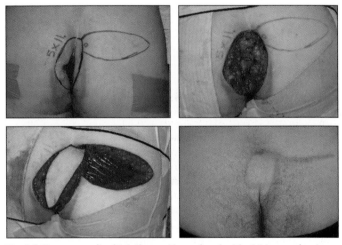

Top left: Recurrent pilonidal disease (the patient had had 14 operations); perforator based flap is marked; the circle indicates the site of the perforator. Top right: Defect after excision to sacral fascia. Bottom left: Flap transposed into defect. Bottom right: Disease-free one year after surgery

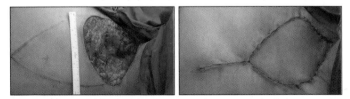

Defect after hidradenitis excision closed by an islanded V-Y flap based on perforating vessels from the thoracodorsal artery

Further reading

- Hasham S, Matteucci P, Stanley PRW, Hart NB. Necrotising fasciitis. *BMJ* 2005;330:830-3.
- Leaper DJ, Harding KG, eds. *Wounds: biology and management.* Oxford: Oxford University Press, 1998.
- McGregor AD, McGregor IA. *Fundamental techniques of plastic surgery, and their surgical applications.* 10th ed. London: Churchill Livingstone, 2000.
- Téot L, Banwell PE, Ziegler UE, eds. *Surgery in wounds.* Berlin: Springer, 2004.

9 Wound dressings

Vanessa Jones, Joseph E Grey, Keith G Harding

Traditionally wet-to-dry gauze has been used to dress wounds. Dressings that create and maintain a moist environment, however, are now considered to provide the optimal conditions for wound healing. Moisture under occlusive dressings not only increases the rate of epithelialisation but also promotes healing through moisture itself and the presence initially of a low oxygen tension (promoting the inflammatory phase). Gauze does not exhibit these properties; it may be disruptive to the healing wound as it dries and cause tissue damage when it is removed. It is not now widely used in the United Kingdom.

Occlusive dressings are thought to increase cell proliferation and activity by retaining an optimum level of wound exudate, which contains vital proteins and cytokines produced in response to injury. These facilitate autolytic debridement of the wound and promote healing. Concerns of increased risk of infection under occlusive dressings have not been substantiated in clinical trials. This article describes wound dressings currently available in the UK.

Low adherent dressings

Low adherent dressings are cheap and widely available. Their major function is to allow exudate to pass through into a secondary dressing while maintaining a moist wound bed.

Most are manufactured in the form of tulles, which are open weave cloth soaked in soft paraffin or chlorhexidine; textiles; or multilayered or perforated plastic films.

They are designed to reduce adherence at the wound bed and are particularly useful for patients with sensitive or fragile skin.

Semipermeable films

Semipermeable films were one of the first major advances in wound management and heralded a major change in the way wounds were managed. They consist of sterile plastic sheets of polyurethane coated with hypoallergenic acrylic adhesive and are used mainly as a transparent primary wound cover.

Although they are impermeable to fluids and bacteria, they are permeable to air and water vapour, the control of which is dependent on the moisture and vapour transmission rate, which varies depending on the brand. It is through this mechanism that this dressing creates a moist wound environment.

Films are very flexible and are good for wounds on "difficult" anatomical sites—for example, over joints. They are unable to cope with large amounts of exudate, however, and may cause maceration of the skin surrounding the wound bed if they are used injudiciously.

Hydrocolloids

Sodium carboxymethylcellulose, gelatin, pectin, elastomers, and adhesives are bonded to a carrier of semipermeable film or a foam sheet to produce a flat, occlusive, adhesive dressing that forms a gel on the wound surface, promoting moist wound healing. Cross linkage of the materials used influences the viscosity of the gel under the dressing. This gel, which may be yellow and malodorous, may be mistaken for infection by the

---

> **Modern dressing technology is based on the principle of creating and maintaining a moist wound environment**

Characteristics of the ideal dressing

- Capable of maintaining a high humidity at the wound site while removing excess exudate
- Free of particles and toxic wound contaminants
- Non-toxic and non-allergenic
- Capable of protecting the wound from further trauma
- Can be removed without causing trauma to the wound
- Impermeable to bacteria
- Thermally insulating
- Will allow gaseous exchange
- Comfortable and conformable
- Require only infrequent changes
- Cost effective
- Long shelf life

Low adherent dressings—suitable for use on flat, shallow wounds with low exudates

Tulles—Bactigras, Jelonet, Paranet, Paratulle, Tullegras, Unitulle, Urgotul

Textiles—Atrauman, Mepilex, Mepitel, NA Dressing, NA Ultra, Tegapore, Tricotex

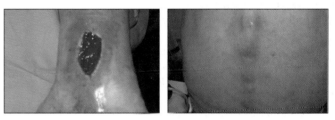

Left: Healthy venous leg ulcer suitable for dressing with low adherent dressing. Right: Wound suitable for dressing with semipermeable film

---

Semipermeable films

Examples include Bioclusive, Mefilm, OpSite Flexigrid,* OpSite Plus, Tegaderm

- Suitable for flat, shallow wounds with low to medium exudates
- Promote moist environment
- Adhere to healthy skin but not to wound
- Allow visual checks
- May be left in place several days
- Useful as secondary dressing
- Provide no cushioning
- Not for infected or heavily exuding wounds

*Not available on prescription in UK primary care.

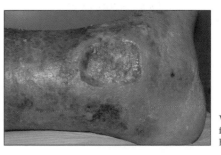

Venous leg ulcer suitable for dressing with hydrocolloid

unwary. Hydrocolloids are virtually impermeable to water vapour and air and can be used to rehydrate dry necrotic eschar and promote autolytic debridement. They are reported to reduce wound pain, and their barrier properties allow the patient to bathe or shower and continue with normal daily activities without disturbing or risking contamination of the wound. Caution should be exercised when using hydrocolloids for wounds that require frequent inspection—for example, for diabetic foot ulcers.

Hydrocolloid fibres are now available in the form of a hydrophilic, non-woven flat sheet, referred to as hydrofibre dressings. On contact with exudate, fibres are converted from a dry dressing to a soft coherent gel sheet, making them suitable for wounds with a large amount of exudate.

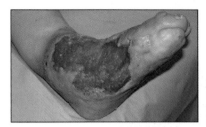

Foot wound complicated by heterotopic calcification suitable for dressing with hydrofibres

Hydrocolloid dressings (including hydrofibres)

Type of dressing	Uses
Hydrocolloid sheets: Alione, CombiDERM, CombiDERM N, Comfeel,* Comfeel Plus, Cutinova Thin,* DuoDERM Extra Thin,* Granuflex,* Tegasorb, Tegasorb Thin	Cavity or flat shallow wounds with low to medium exudate; absorbent; conformable; good in "difficult" areas—heel, elbow, sacrum
Hydrocolloid paste: GranuGel Paste*	May be left in place for several days; useful debriding agent; may cause maceration
Hydrofibre: Aquacel (Hydrofibre), Versiva	Useful in flat wounds, cavities, sinuses, undermining wounds; medium to high exudate wounds; highly absorbent; non-adherent; may be left in place for several days; needs secondary dressing

*Not available on prescription in UK primary care.

> **Hydrocolloid fibres (hydrofibres) are often used on wounds where, traditionally, alginates have been used**

Hydrogels

Hydrogels consist of a matrix of insoluble polymers with up to 96% water content enabling them to donate water molecules to the wound surface and to maintain a moist environment at the wound bed. As the polymers are only partially hydrated, hydrogels have the ability to absorb a degree of wound exudate, the amount varying between different brands. They transmit moisture vapour and oxygen, but their bacterial and fluid permeability is dependent on the type of secondary dressing used.

Hydrogels promote wound debridement by rehydration of non-viable tissue, thus facilitating the process of natural autolysis. Amorphous hydrogels are the most commonly used and are thick, viscous gels.

Hydrogels are considered to be a standard form of management for sloughy or necrotic wounds. They are not indicated for wounds producing high levels of exudate or where there is evidence of gangrenous tissue, which should be kept dry to reduce the risk of infection.

Hydrogels

Examples include Aquaform, Intrasite, GranuGel, Nu-Gel, Purilon, Sterigel
- Supply moisture to wounds with low to medium exudate
- Suitable for sloughy or necrotic wounds
- Useful in flat wounds, cavities, and sinuses
- May be left in place several days
- Need secondary dressing
- May cause maceration

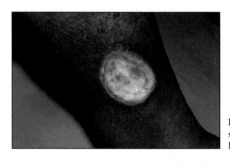

Dry, sloughy leg wound suitable for dressing with hydrogel

Alginates

Alginates are produced from the naturally occurring calcium and sodium salts of alginic acid found in a family of brown seaweed (Phaeophyceae). They generally fall into one of two kinds: those containing 100% calcium alginate or those that contain a combination of calcium with sodium alginate, usually in a ratio of 80:20.

Alginates are rich in either mannuronic acid or guluronic acid, the relative amount of each influencing the amount of exudate absorbed and the shape the dressing will retain. Alginates partly dissolve on contact with wound fluid to form a hydrophilic gel as a result of the exchange of sodium ions in wound fluid for calcium ions in the dressing. Those high in mannuronic acid (such as Kaltostat) can be washed off the wound easily with saline, but those high in guluronic acid (such as Sorbsan) tend to retain their basic structure and should be removed from the wound bed in one piece.

Alginates can absorb 15 to 20 times their weight of fluid, making them suitable for highly exuding wounds. They should

Alginates

Examples include Algisite, Algosteril, Kaltostat,* Melgisorb, SeaSorb, Sorbsan, Sorbsan SA,* Tegagen, Urgosorb
- Useful in cavities and sinuses, and for undermining wounds
- For all wound types with high exudates
- Highly absorbent
- Need secondary dressing
- Need to be changed daily

*Not available on prescription in UK primary care

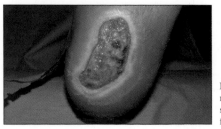

Diabetic foot ulcer with maceration to surrounding skin suitable for dressing with alginate

not be used, however, on wounds with little or no exudate as they will adhere to the healing wound surface, causing pain and damaging healthy tissue on removal.

Foam dressings

Foam dressings are manufactured as either a polyurethane or silicone foam. They transmit moisture vapour and oxygen and provide thermal insulation to the wound bed. Polyurethane foams consist of two or three layers, including a hydrophilic wound contact surface and a hydrophobic backing, making them highly absorbent. They facilitate uniform dispersion of exudate throughout the absorbent layer and prevent exterior leakage (strike-through) due to the presence of a semipermeable backing.

Polyurethane foam dressings are also available as a cavity dressing—small chips of hydrophilic polyurethane foam enclosed in a membrane of perforated polymeric film, giving a loosely filled bag.

Silicone foams consist of a polymer of silicone elastomer derived from two liquids, which, when mixed together, form a foam while expanding to fit the wound shape forming a soft open-cell foam dressing. The major advantage of foam is the ability to contain exudate. In addition, silicone foam dressings protect the area around the wound from further damage.

Antimicrobial dressings

Silver, in ionic or nanocrystalline form, has for many years been used as an antimicrobial agent particularly in the treatment of burns (in the form of silver sulfadiazine cream). The recent development of dressings impregnated with silver has widened its use for many other wound types that are either colonised or infected.

Iodine also has the ability to lower the microbiological load in chronic wounds. Clinically it is mainly used in one of two formats: (a) as povidone-iodine (polyvinylpyrrolidone-iodine complex), an iodophor (a compound of iodine linked to a non-ionic surfactant), which is produced as an impregnated tulle; and (b) as cadexomer iodine (a three dimensional starch lattice containing 0.9% iodine). Cadexomer iodine has good absorptive properties: 1 g of cadexomer iodine can absorb up to 7 ml of fluid. As fluid is absorbed, iodine is slowly released, reducing the bacterial load and also debriding the wound of debris. This mode of action facilitates the delivery of iodine over a prolonged period of time—thus, in theory, maintaining a constant level of iodine in the wound bed.

Caution is required in patients with a thyroid disease owing to possible systemic uptake of iodine. For this reason, thyroid function should be monitored in patients who are treated with iodine dressings.

Metronidazole gel is often used for the control of odour caused by anaerobic bacteria. This is particularly useful in the management of fungating malignant wounds. It may be used alone or as an adjunct to other dressings.

Unwanted effects of dressings

Maceration of the skin surrounding a wound may occur if a dressing with a low absorptive capacity is used on a heavily exuding wound. If the dressing is highly absorptive then more frequent dressing changes may be needed, in addition to investigation and management of the cause of the exudate (such as infection).

> The ion exchange properties of some alginates make them useful haemostatic agents, and as such they are particularly useful for postoperative wound packing

---

Foam dressings

Type of dressing	Uses
Adhesive sheets: Allevyn Adhesive, Allevyn Lite Island, Allevyn Thin, Allevyn Plus Adhesive, Biatain Adhesive, Lyofoam Extra Adhesive, Tielle Plus, Tielle Lite, Tielle	Flat, shallow wounds (control of exudate depending on type of foam); give degree of cushioning; may be left in place for two to three days
Non-adherent sheets: Allevyn,* Allevyn Lite, Lyofoam,* Lyofoam Extra*	Need secondary dressing
Allevyn Cavity, Allevyn Plus Cavity, Cavi-Care	Cavity wound with medium to high exudate

*Not available on prescription in UK primary care.

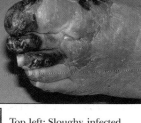

Venous leg ulceration in background of chronic oedema suitable for dressing with foam

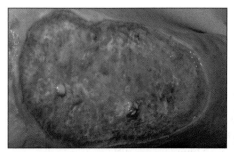

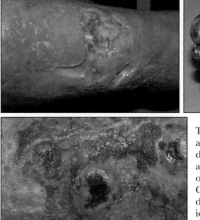

Top left: Sloughy, infected arterial ulcer suitable for dressing with compound antimicrobial dressing (silver or iodine based). Top right: Gangrenous foot suitable for dressing with antimicrobial iodine impregnated dressing. Left: Malodorous malignant melanoma ulcer suitable for treatment with topical metronidazole

---

Antimicrobial dressings

For use in all locally infected wounds
- Acticoat
- Actisorb Silver 200
- Aquacel Ag
- Arglaes
- Avance
- Inadine
- Iodoflex
- Iodosorb
- Metrotop Gel

> Inappropriate use of dressings may lead to unwanted effects

ABC of wound healing

The skin surrounding a highly exuding wound may be further protected through the use of emollients (such as 50:50 mix of white soft paraffin and liquid paraffin) or the application of barrier films (such as Cavilon). Conversely, use of a highly absorptive dressing on a dry wound may lead to disruption of healthy tissue on the wound surface and cause pain when removed.

Allergic reactions are not uncommon: the dressing should be avoided, and the allergy may need to be treated with potent topical steroids. Tapes used to keep dressings in place are common causes of allergy. Many dressings require secondary dressings—for example, padding on highly exuding wounds—which may make them bulky. Secondary dressings should not be too tight, especially on patients with peripheral vascular disease.

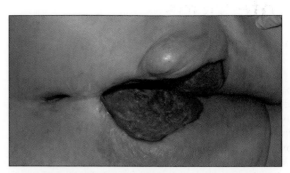

Abdominoperineal resection wound treated with vacuum assisted closure. The skin edges are protected with a barrier cream to prevent maceration

Further reading

- Choucair M, Phillips T. A review of wound healing and dressings material. *Skin and Aging* 1998;6:(suppl):37-43.
- Hermans MH, Bolton LL. Air exposure versus occlusion: merits and disadvantages of different dressings. *J Wound Care* 1993;2:362-5.
- Morgan DA. Wound management products in the drug tariff. *Pharmaceutical Journal* 1999;263:820-5.
- Thomas S, Leigh IM. Wound dressings. In: Leaper DJ, Harding KG, eds. *Wounds: biology and management.* Oxford: Oxford University Press, 1998:166-83.
- Turner TD. Development of wound management products in chronic wound care. In: Krasner D, Rodeheaver G, Sibbald RG, eds. *Chronic wound care: a clinical source book for healthcare professionals.* 3rd ed. Wayne, PA: HMP Communications, 2001.
- Winter G. Formation of scab and the rate of epithelialisation of superficial wounds in the skin of the young domestic pig. *Nature* 1962;193:293-4.
- Vermeulen H, Ubbink D, Goossens A, de Vos R, Legemate D. Dressings and topical agents for surgical wounds healing by secondary intention. *Cochrane Database Syst Rev* 2005;(4):CD003554.

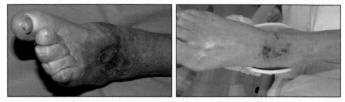

Left: Allergy to dressing used to treat arterial leg ulceration. Note erythematous skin with sharply demarcated edges corresponding to the shape of the offending dressing. Right: Ulceration over the anterior aspect of the ankle caused by inappropriately tight bandage

10 Infections

Brendan Healy, Andrew Freedman

Despite optimal treatment some wounds are slow to heal. The challenge clinically and microbiologically is to identify those wounds in which healing is impaired as a result of infection or heavy bacterial burden and in which systemic or topical antimicrobial treatment will be of benefit.

Staphylococci and streptococci are the most commonly encountered pathogenic organisms in community acquired superficial wounds. More unusual organisms may be found in bite wounds, and these reflect the source of the bite. Pathogenic organisms causing surgical wound infections vary according to the anatomical site of surgery. Antibiotic resistant organisms, such as methicillin resistant *Staphylococcus aureus* (MRSA), are more commonly encountered, reflecting the hospital flora.

When to sample

It is inappropriate to swab all wounds: swabs should be taken only from overtly infected wounds and from wounds that are deteriorating, increasing in size, or failing to make satisfactory progress despite an optimal environment for wound healing. Indicators of wound infection include redness, swelling, purulent exudate, smell, pain, and systemic illness in the absence of other foci. Subtle signs of local wound infection include unhealthy "foamy" granulation tissue, contact bleeding, tissue breakdown, and epithelial bridging.

Types of sample

Superficial wound swabs—The ease of obtaining and processing superficial wound swabs, combined with their relatively low cost and non-invasive nature, make them in most instances the most appropriate method for wound sampling. Organisms cultured from a superficial swab may, however, simply reflect the colonising bacterial flora and are not always representative of the pathogenic organisms invading deeper tissue. This is particularly relevant to deep surgical and deep penetrating wounds in which infection from internal sources may occur.

Tissue and pus—Tissue or pus, or both, should be collected whenever possible, as growth from these samples is more representative of pathogenic flora. These are amenable to quantitative microbiological analysis and other techniques used to improve the diagnostic yield. Tissue biopsy should always be carried out when therapeutic debridement of the wound is done, in cases of osteomyelitis, and when superficial sampling methods have been ineffective.

Less invasive techniques—Less invasive sampling techniques—such as dermabrasion and various absorbent pads—have been developed. A wide range of products is available, but no single method is used routinely yet.

Microbiological analysis

Semiquantitative analysis
Most laboratories will perform a semiquantitative analysis on wound swabs. This entails grading bacterial growth as scanty, light, moderate, or heavy. Semiquantitative analysis introduces a bias towards motile and fast growing organisms.

Infection is a major source of failed wound healing

Management of bite wounds

- Carry out meticulous surgical debridement and cleansing of wound
- Send deep tissue specimens for microbiology testing
- Consider empirical treatment with antibiotics
- Consider tetanus prophylaxis
- Seek microbiological advice if bite was by exotic animal

Signs of wound infection

- Redness
- Heat
- Pain
- Swelling
- Exudate (purulent, serous, or serosanguinous)
- Odour
- Poor healing
- Contact bleeding
- Epithelial bridging
- Tissue breakdown
- Presence of unhealthy granulation tissue
- Systemic illness in the absence of other focus of infection

---

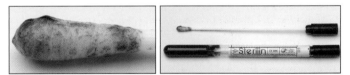

A charcoal swab preserves bacteria during transport to the laboratory

---

How to take a superficial wound swab

- Removal of superficial debris followed by swabbing of the wound bed is considered to be the best way to obtain a superficial wound swab
- Swabs containing transport media and charcoal should be used as they help to preserve bacteria before laboratory analysis
- Timely delivery of the swab to the microbiology laboratory is essential

---

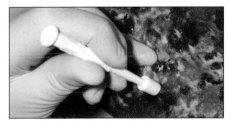

Punch biopsy for microbiological analysis

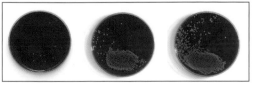

Semiquantitative analysis of swab showing light or scanty, moderate, and heavy growth of *Staphylococcus aureus*

Fastidious organisms such as anaerobes may be under-represented. Semiquantitative counts have been shown to correlate with quantitative tissue counts in both burn wounds and diabetic foot ulcers.

> **Superficial wound swabs are not always representative of the pathogenic organisms invading deeper tissue**

Microbiological analysis

Type of analysis	Suitable samples	Advantages	Disadvantages
Gram stain	Tissue, pus, or swab transported immediately to laboratory	Instant results; good correlation with quantitative counts	Poor sensitivity; no antibiotic sensitivity pattern
Quantitative culture	Tissue, pus, dermabrasion specimens, absorbent pad specimens	Counts $> 10^5$ organisms or colony forming units per gram of tissue predict wound infection	Invasive; labour intensive; costly
Semiquantitative culture	All specimens	Practical; can be carried out on swab specimens; some correlation with quantitative analysis	Imprecise; bias towards motile/fast growing organisms; sampling of superficial colonising bacteria

Quantitative analysis

Bacterial load greater than 100 000 organisms or colony forming units per gram of tissue or mm^3 of pus is a predictor of wound infection.

However, some wounds that are more heavily colonised will heal spontaneously, and, conversely, some organisms are able to cause serious infection at much lower levels of colonisation. Infection depends on the pathogenicity of the organism, the type of wound, and the host response.

Interpretation of results

Most wound swabs will yield bacterial growth. Growth of bacteria from wounds is not synonymous with infection, and treatment based on microbiological results alone is not warranted.

Treatment

Wound infections in association with systemic illness, deep invasion, or cellulitis require empirical systemic antibiotic treatment while culture results are awaited. Choice of treatment will depend on factors such as the type and site of wound; previous microbiological results; and host factors such as drug allergies. Clinicians must always be alert to the possibility of necrotising fasciitis. A high level of suspicion followed by prompt aggressive surgical debridement of devitalised necrotic tissue is essential if the patient is to survive. Important clinical markers include pain disproportionate to clinical signs, anaesthesia over the infected area, and systemic illness.

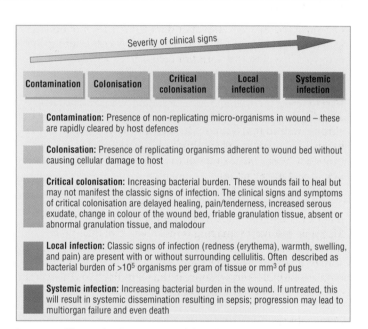

Severity of clinical signs →

| Contamination | Colonisation | Critical colonisation | Local infection | Systemic infection |

Contamination: Presence of non-replicating micro-organisms in wound – these are rapidly cleared by host defences

Colonisation: Presence of replicating organisms adherent to wound bed without causing cellular damage to host

Critical colonisation: Increasing bacterial burden. These wounds fail to heal but may not manifest the classic signs of infection. The clinical signs and symptoms of critical colonisation are delayed healing, pain/tenderness, increased serous exudate, change in colour of the wound bed, friable granulation tissue, absent or abnormal granulation tissue, and malodour

Local infection: Classic signs of infection (redness (erythema), warmth, swelling, and pain) are present with or without surrounding cellulitis. Often described as bacterial burden of >10^5 organisms per gram of tissue or mm^3 of pus

Systemic infection: Increasing bacterial burden in the wound. If untreated, this will result in systemic dissemination resulting in sepsis; progression may lead to multiorgan failure and even death

Spectrum of interaction between bacteria and host

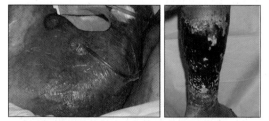

Left: Extensive cellulitis complicating laparotomy wound. Right: Severely locally infected wound showing unhealthy granulation tissue

Empirical antibiotic treatment of wound infection in systemically unwell patient*

Type of wound	Antibiotic
Wound infection	Co-amoxiclav
Surgical wound infection	Cefuroxime and metronidazole or co-amoxiclav
Bite wound	Co-amoxiclav
Diabetic ulcer	Co-amoxiclav and ciprofloxacin
Osteomyelitis	Co-amoxiclav or ciprofloxacin and clindamycin
Necrotising fasciitis	High dose benzylpenicillin plus clindamycin (with or without ciprofloxacin)
MRSA infection suspected	Vancomycin or linezolid

*Rough guide only. In general, treatment should be guided by discussion with the local microbiology department. Choice of antibiotics will depend on previous microbiology where available, previous antibiotic treatment, site of surgery, and the local prevalence of MRSA.

Clinical markers of necrotising fasciitis*

Early presentation
- Pain (may be disproportionate to clinical signs)
- Cellulitis
- Swelling of the affected region
- Induration
- Skin anaesthesia
- Fever
- Tachycardia

Late presentation
- Severe pain
- Skin discoloration (purple or black)
- Blistering
- Haemorrhagic bullae
- Crepitus
- Discharge of "dishwater" fluid
- Severe sepsis or systemic inflammatory response syndrome
- Multiorgan failure

*From Hasham et al, 2005 (see Further Reading box)

Treatment of locally infected wounds with topical antiseptics such as silver compounds or iodine will be sufficient in most instances. Topical treatment avoids the potential side effects of systemic antibiotics, such as *Clostridium difficile* diarrhoea, anaphylaxis, gastrointestinal upset, and, perhaps most importantly, selection of resistant organisms. Systemic treatment may be indicated if topical medication is unsuccessful.

In general, topical antibiotics are not recommended. Reasons for this include inadequate penetration for deep skin infections, development of antibiotic resistance, hypersensitivity reactions, systemic absorption when applied to large wounds, and local irritant effects leading to further delay in wound healing. Short courses of silver sulfadiazine or topical metronidazole can be useful, however, in certain circumstances—for example, with burns and chronic ulcers.

Osteomyelitis associated with wound infection

Osteomyelitis may develop after direct inoculation of bone from a contiguous focus of infection. This can be a devastating complication of wound infection, requiring specialist intervention and management.

Diagnosis

The diagnosis of osteomyelitis should be considered in any chronic wound that does not heal despite optimal treatment or in any wound (especially in those with diabetes) that can be probed to bone. Plain x rays of the affected area should be the first line of investigation.

Radiographic changes, however, can lag behind the evolution of infection by at least two weeks; a single, negative plain x ray film does not, therefore, exclude osteomyelitis. Magnetic resonance imaging is more sensitive than plain radiography. Nuclear scintigraphy—either a technetium bone scan or a labelled white cell scan—may also be helpful but requires careful interpretation. It can be difficult to differentiate osteomyelitis from chronic soft tissue infection.

Management

Antibiotics penetrate poorly into devitalised bone, and long courses of antibiotics may be required. It is therefore important to define the infecting organism(s) from the outset so that antibiotic treatment can be targeted. Ideally, in the absence of systemic illness, antibiotics should not be started before microbiological sampling of the infected bone.

Surgery followed by prolonged intravenous antibiotic treatment (generally a minimum of six weeks), is indicated in selected patients. Periodic antibiotic treatment at times of wound deterioration or of systemic illness may be appropriate if cure is unachievable.

Surgery

Surgery enables debridement of all necrotic bone and tissue and provides deep samples for microbiological analysis. In some patients, surgery is not possible either because of the site of the wound or because of the patient's debility. Under these circumstances, a prolonged course of antibiotics may be warranted.

Antibiotic treatment

Choice of treatment is dependent on the antibiotic sensitivity pattern of the infecting organism(s) along with antibiotic properties, such as bone penetration, and host factors, such as drug allergy. Combination therapy is often used to gain maximal effect. Inflammatory markers (including C reactive

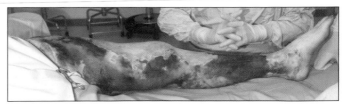

Necrotising fasciitis

Topical antimicrobial preparations

- Iodine releasing agents (povidone-iodine preparations, cadexomer-iodine preparations)
- Potassium permanganate solution
- Silver releasing agents (composite silver dressings, silver sulfadiazine)
- Topical antibiotic (metronidazole)

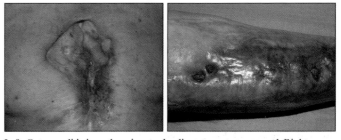

Left: Osteomyelitis in a chronic, non-healing sternotomy wound. Right: Osteomyelitis arising at the site of a previous traumatic wound to the tibia, previously healed by reconstructive surgery. The sinuses probe to bone

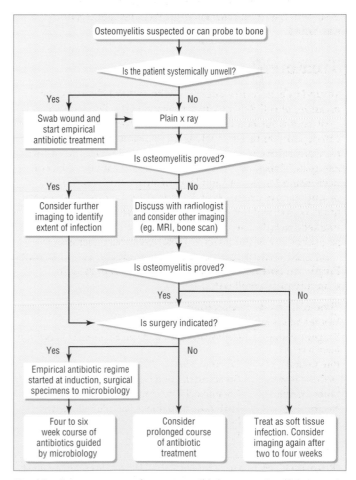

Algorithm for management when osteomyelitis is suspected or if the wound can be probed to bone

protein and erythrocyte sedimentation rate) and radiological images can be used to monitor response.

Methicillin resistant *Staphylococcus aureus*

The incidence of MRSA wound infection and osteomyelitis is increasing. Isolation of MRSA from a wound, however, does not require treatment in the absence of clinical signs of infection. Topical antimicrobial agents, such as iodine and silver compounds, have activity against MRSA and may be used in localised wound infection when there is no evidence of invasion, cellulitis, or systemic upset.

In a systemically unwell individual, a glycopeptide (vancomycin or teicoplanin) should be administered. In all cases of MRSA osteomyelitis and in some MRSA wound infections a second antistaphylococcal agent with good penetration to bone and superficial skin sites should be added—for example, fusidic acid or rifampicin. Both rifampicin and fusidic acid can cause hepatitis and require regular monitoring of liver function tests.

With the exception of linezolid, evidence for the use of oral antibiotics in MRSA infections is lacking. However, when oral antibiotics are used, combinations are recommended to protect against the development of resistance. Combinations of rifampicin or fusidic acid with either trimethoprim or minocycline have been used with some success. The combination of rifampicin with fusidic acid is not advisable because of the increased risk of hepatotoxicity.

Linezolid, an oxazolidinone, is a new agent active against MRSA. It has excellent bioavailability, can be administered orally, and has good skin and bone penetration. Linezolid is generally well tolerated, but can cause bone marrow suppression, and regular haematological monitoring is therefore required. Linezolid use is currently limited by its high cost.

Agents that may be available in the near future include daptomycin, tigecycline, and dalbavancin.

The figure showing the spectrum of interaction between bacteria and host was supplied by J E Grey and Stuart Enoch.

Radiological improvement will often lag behind clinical improvement by up to six weeks

Further reading

- Hasham S, Matteucci P, Stanley PR, Hart NB. Necrotising fasciitis. *BMJ* 2005;330:830-3.
- Weigelt J, Itani K, Stevens D, Lau W, Dryden M, Knirsch C, Linezolid CSSTI Study Group. Linezolid versus vancomycin in treatment of complicated skin and soft tissue infections. *Antimicrob Agents Chemother* 2005;49:2260-6.
- Eron LJ, Lipsky BA, Low DE, Nathwani D, Tice AD, Volturo GA, Expert Panel on Managing Skin and Soft Tissue Infections. Managing skin and soft tissue infections: expert panel recommendations on key decision points. *J Antimicrob Chemother* 2003;52(suppl 1):i3-17.
- Bisno AL, Cockerill FR 3rd, Bermudez CT. The initial outpatient-physician encounter in group A streptococcal necrotizing fasciitis. *Clin Infect Dis* 2000;31:607-8.

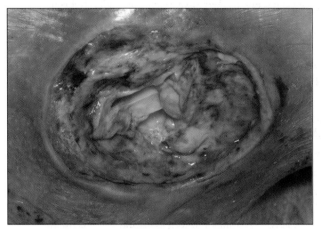

Pressure sore associated with MRSA osteomyelitis. Bone is visible at the base of the ulcer

11   Non-surgical and drug treatments

Stuart Enoch, Joseph E Grey, Keith G Harding

Despite great strides in technological innovations and the emergence of a wide range of treatments for wounds, non-healing wounds continue to perplex and challenge doctors. Various non-surgical approaches have been developed and numerous drugs have been introduced to aid the management of such wounds.

Non-surgical treatments

Bandages and hosiery
Compression bandages are used to treat lower limb ulcers secondary to venous insufficiency (venous leg ulcers) and lymphoedema. Single layer compression bandages (elastic) are classified into four groups according to the predetermined levels of compression they provide at the ankle. Inelastic compression bandages (short stretch), when applied at full extension, improve the calf muscle pump action and exert higher pressures when the patient is upright (and walking) and lower pressures at rest. They are useful in patients who are adequately mobile. An elasticated tubular bandage (one to three layers) may be useful to treat and prevent venous leg ulcers.

Single layer compression bandages

Class (level of compression)	Indication	Examples
3a (light (14-17 mm Hg))	To treat simple VLU	Elset, Litepress
3b (moderate (18-24 mm Hg))	To treat VLU and ulcers secondary to lymphoedema	Tensoplus Forte, Coban
3c (high (25-35 mm Hg))	As for class 3b plus gross varicose veins in moderate sized legs	Tensopres, Setopress, Surepress
3d (extra-high (36-50 mm Hg))	To treat extensive VLU, ulcers secondary to lymphoedema, extensive varicose veins, and post-thrombotic venous insufficiency in patients with very large and oedematous legs	Elastic web bandages (blue line or red line webbing)

VLU = venous leg ulcer.

Multilayer compression bandaging, such as the four layer method, is well established in the management of venous leg ulcers. It consists of four layers—padding, a crepe bandage, and classes 3a and 3b (UK classification) compression bandages—applied from the base of the toes to knee. Ideally, it should be left in place for four to seven days. Although effective, the bulkiness of these layers may lead to non-compliance in some patients. Its use is limited in heavily exuding ulcers as repeated dressing changes may be needed.

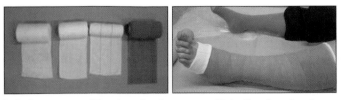

Left: Components of four layer bandage system. Right: Four layer bandage system to treat venous ulcer (note class II compression stocking on right leg for prevention of ulceration)

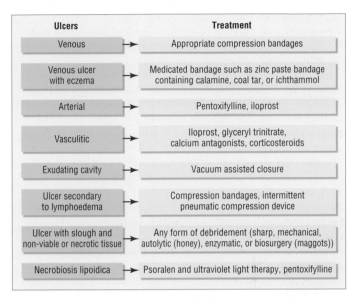

Ulcers	Treatment
Venous	Appropriate compression bandages
Venous ulcer with eczema	Medicated bandage such as zinc paste bandage containing calamine, coal tar, or ichthammol
Arterial	Pentoxifylline, iloprost
Vasculitic	Iloprost, glyceryl trinitrate, calcium antagonists, corticosteroids
Exudating cavity	Vacuum assisted closure
Ulcer secondary to lymphoedema	Compression bandages, intermittent pneumatic compression device
Ulcer with slough and non-viable or necrotic tissue	Any form of debridement (sharp, mechanical, autolytic (honey), enzymatic, or biosurgery (maggots))
Necrobiosis lipoidica	Psoralen and ultraviolet light therapy, pentoxifylline

Non-surgical and drug treatments to consider in the treatment of chronic ulcers

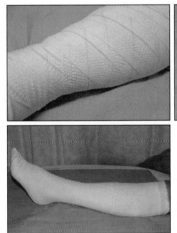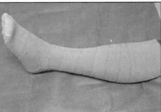

Top left: Single layer elastic compression bandage. Top right: Inelastic (short stretch) compression bandage. Left: Three layer elasticated tubular bandage

Caution in use of compression bandages
- Appropriate clinical evaluation is essential before using any form of compression treatment
- Injudicious use may lead to serious complications, including limb gangrene
- Distal circulation of the limb should be carefully assessed and peripheral vascular disease excluded
- Caution should be exercised in patients with peripheral neuropathy

Graduated compression hosiery (UK classes I to III) is primarily used to prevent recurrence of venous leg ulcers and to control symptoms associated with varicose veins. The use of compression hosiery below the knee is associated with increased patient adherence

Medicated bandages such as zinc paste bandages can be useful in treating some leg ulcers. They can be left undisturbed for up to a week. A zinc paste bandage containing calamine, coal tar, or ichthammol can be used if there is associated venous eczema. Medicated bandages provide no compression.

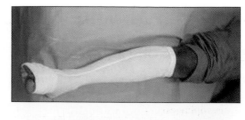

Medicated bandage

Intermittent pneumatic compression

Intermittent pneumatic compression is effective in treating longstanding venous leg ulcers associated with severe oedema that are refractory to conventional compression therapy alone.

Intermittent pneumatic compression provides compression (range 20-120 mm Hg) at preset intervals (average 70 seconds) through an electrically inflatable "boot" of variable lengths. It is generally used two hours a day for up to six weeks. It improves venous and lymphatic flow and is useful in patients with comorbidities that limit mobility. It should be used as an adjunct to, rather than a substitute for, conventional compression therapy. Care should be taken in patients with cardiac failure.

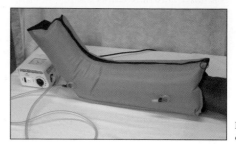

Intermittent pneumatic compression device

Vacuum assisted closure

Vacuum assisted closure is a non-invasive, negative pressure healing technique that is used to treat a wide range of chronic, non-healing wounds.

The vacuum assisted closure device uses controlled subatmospheric pressure to remove excess wound fluid from the extravascular space, leading to improved local oxygenation and peripheral blood flow. This promotes angiogenesis and formation of granulation tissue, which are particularly useful in deep cavitating wounds to expedite "filling" of the wound space.

Vacuum assisted closure is contraindicated in patients with thin, easily bruised or abraded skin and in those with neoplasms as part of the wound floor. Cost and patient adherence may be issues of concern in some cases.

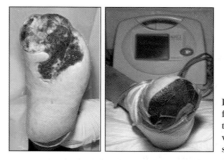

Diabetic foot ulcer suitable for vacuum assisted closure therapy (far left) and vacuum assisted closure in situ (left).

Hyperbaric oxygen

The use of hyperbaric oxygen has been recommended as an adjunctive therapy to treat a variety of non-healing wounds (as many non-healing tissues are hypoxic). Treatment is given by increasing the atmospheric pressure in a chamber while the patient is breathing 100% oxygen. Side effects such as seizures and pneumothorax have been reported with hyperbaric oxygen.

A systematic review of the Cochrane database, however, has found insufficient evidence for its effectiveness in healing chronic wounds, although it might have a role in reducing the risk of major amputation in patients with diabetic foot ulcers (see third article this series).

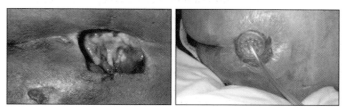

Left: Grade 4 sacral pressure ulcer suitable for vacuum assisted closure therapy. Right: Vacuum assisted closure in situ

Further rigorous randomised controlled trials are necessary to ascertain the type of ulcers that may benefit from treatment with hyperbaric oxygen

Biosurgery (myiasis)

Biosurgery uses sterile maggots (usually of the green bottle fly, *Lucilia sericata*), which digest sloughy and necrotic material from wounds without damaging the surrounding healthy tissue.

They have been shown in small scale trials to be useful in the treatment of venous, arterial, and pressure ulcers. Some patients complain of increased pain in the wound, and psychological discomfort and aesthetics may be issues for some individuals.

Other approaches

Other non-surgical approaches that have a scientific basis and thus have been advocated in the treatment of chronic wounds include radiant heat dressing, ultrasound therapy, laser treatment, hydrotherapy, electrotherapy, electromagnetic therapy, and PUVA therapy (psoralen plus ultraviolet A irradiation).

However, few randomised controlled trials have studied the effectiveness of these treatments.

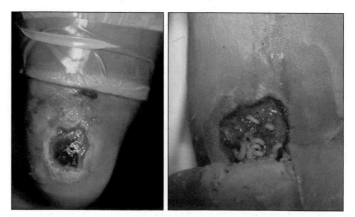

Left: Pressure ulcer before debridement with larval (maggot) therapy. Right: The same ulcer 12 days after debridement with larval therapy (with maggots in situ)

Non-surgical approaches that have been advocated for treating chronic wounds

Type	Mechanism of action/principle	Wound type	Evidence; current status
Radiant heat dressing	Improves tissue oxygenation and increases subcutaneous oxygen tension	Mainly postoperative wounds; diabetic ulcers; pressure ulcers	Limited evidence; not in routine use
Ultrasound therapy	Mechanical effect causing micromassage of tissue; anti-inflammatory effect (due to reduction in macrophages)	Pressure ulcers and VLU	Limited evidence; not in routine use
Laser	Stimulates fibroblast activity and collagen metabolism; promotes neovascularisation; inhibits inflammation	VLU, diabetic ulcers, and burns	Limited evidence; not in routine use
Hydrotherapy	Form of mechanical debridement; removes loosely attached devitalised tissue and other cellular debris from wound bed	Pressure ulcers, VLU, and other chronic wounds containing excess slough or necrotic tissue	Practised in USA, but not well established in UK
Electrotherapy	Stimulates body's endogenous bioelectric system by delivering therapeutic levels of electric current into wound	TENS* is used to treat some ischaemic ulcers, diabetic foot ulcer, and pressure ulcers	Limited evidence; TENS* used in specialist centres
Electromagnetic therapy	Promotes cytokine synthesis in the topically applied mononuclear cells (autologous)	Ischaemic ulcers, pressure ulcers, and VLU	Limited evidence; not in routine use

VLU = venous leg ulcer.
*Form of electrotherapy.

Drugs

Pentoxifylline, a methylxanthine that improves perfusion of peripheral vascular beds, is useful in patients with ulcers secondary to peripheral vascular disease. It improves capillary microcirculation by decreasing blood viscosity and reducing platelet aggregation. It may also inhibit tumour necrosis factor-α, an inflammatory cytokine involved in non-healing wounds. Although mainly indicated for ulcers secondary to peripheral vascular disease, pentoxifylline is useful in patients with venous leg ulcer who cannot tolerate compression or in whom compression is ineffective. It may also be beneficial in rare but complex ulcers such as sickle cell ulcers, livedoid vasculitis, and necrobiosis lipoidica.

Iloprost, a prostacyclin analogue, is an established treatment for intermittent claudication, severe limb ischaemia, and prevention of imminent gangrene, and to reduce the pain and clinical symptoms associated with Raynaud's disease. Intravenous iloprost is useful in promoting healing of arterial ulcers and vasculitic ulcers secondary to connective tissue diseases such as rheumatoid arthritis and scleroderma.

Antimicrobials including iodine based preparations and silver releasing agents are used to treat infected wounds (there may be a dose dependent effect). Antimicrobial agents target bacteria at several level (cell membrane, cytoplasmic organelle, and nucleic acid), thus minimising bacterial resistance. They can be used either on their own or in conjunction with systemic antibiotics. The many silver releasing agents, in dressing form, aim to deliver sustained doses of silver to the wound. In addition to the microbicidal effect of silver on common wound contaminants, silver may also be effective against methicillin resistant *Staphylococcus aureus* (MRSA).

Glyceryl trinitrate, a nitric oxide donor, is effective in the management of chronic anal fissures when applied topically as 0.2% ointment. Nitric oxide causes vasodilatation, and uncontrolled studies have suggested a potential role for glyceryl trinitrate in treating chronic wounds of ischaemic aetiology, including vasculitic ulcers. Headache, sometimes troublesome, is the most commonly encountered side effect with glyceryl trinitrate: lower concentrations may avoid this side effect.

Calcium antagonists such as diltiazem and nifedipine are useful in treating vasculitic ulcers secondary to Raynaud's disease and connective tissue diseases. In Raynaud's disease, they restore blood flow to the digits and thus are useful in treating ulcers and the prevention of necrosis in the extremities.

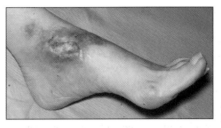

Arterial ulcer suitable for pentoxifylline treatment

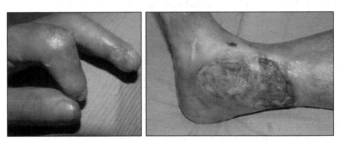

Left: Ulcers secondary to Raynaud's disease suitable for iloprost therapy.
Right: Ulcer secondary to rheumatoid arthritis suitable for iloprost therapy

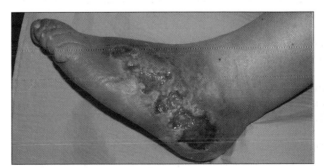

Infected wound suitable for topical antimicrobial therapy

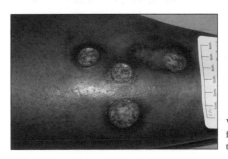

Vasculitic ulcer suitable for treatment with glyceryl trinitrate

41

Systemic corticosteroids are useful in treating ulcers secondary to connective tissue diseases, including rheumatoid arthritis, scleroderma, and other vasculitic disorders. They promote healing by attenuating the excessive inflammatory response. Long term use of corticosteroids, however, may have a detrimental effect on healing. Patients taking long term, high dose steroids should be offered bone protection with bisphosphonates.

Zinc, an antioxidant, used in a paste bandage may be useful in treating infected leg ulcers. Oral zinc sulphate treatment may be beneficial in patients with chronic ulcers who have low serum zinc levels.

Phenytoin, applied topically, promotes wound healing by inhibiting the enzyme collagenase. It is effective in some low grade pressure ulcers and trophic ulcers due to leprosy. The possibility of systemic absorption and toxicity has limited its use.

Retinoids (derived from vitamin A) have an impact on wound healing through their effects on angiogenesis, collagen synthesis, and epithelialisation. Vitamin A is necessary for normal epidermal maintenance. Although the value of retinoids in chronic wounds is unclear, topical tretinoin (0.05-0.1%) has been shown to accelerate re-epithelialisation of dermabraded and chemically peeled wounds in humans, and partial and full thickness wounds in animal models.

Analgesics are needed for many ulcers. They may range from simple analgesics to opiates in individuals whose the pain is severe. Pain from ulcers associated with neuropathy may benefit from treatment with certain tricyclic antidepressants (such as amitriptyline) or antiepileptic drugs (such as gabapentin). Intractable pain may necessitate intervention by specialist pain management teams.

Natural products

Honey, of the pasture and manuka varieties, has some antibacterial action, inhibits excessive inflammatory response, and promotes autolytic debridement. It is available as an impregnated dressing or as a gel. Honey is used in the treatment of a range of chronic wounds. Clinical data to support its widespread use are limited, however, with insufficient evidence on the type of wounds that may benefit and the amount and duration of application required.

Many other natural products—including yoghurt, tea tree oil, and potato peeling—have been used in various parts of the world to treat ulcers with varying degrees of success; controlled studies are lacking.

Drugs and agents that impair healing

Vasoconstrictors, such as nicotine, cocaine, adrenaline (epinephrine) and ergotamine, cause tissue hypoxia by adversely affecting the microcirculation, leading to impaired wound healing. They should be avoided in patients with acute, surgical, or chronic wounds. Little evidence exists to suggest that immunosuppressants and antineoplastic drugs (such as azathioprine, ciclosporin, cyclophosphamide, methotrexate) affect wound healing in humans. Patients taking immunosuppressants, however, have a slightly increased risk of developing malignant ulcers. A biopsy should be taken if an ulcer develops in these patients.

The photos of maggot therapy were provided by Dr S Thomas of Zoobiotic, and the photo of the manuka bush was provided by Dr R Cooper, University of Wales Institute, Cardiff.

Effect of some commonly used drugs on wound healing

Class and name of drug	Effects
NSAIDs Ibuprofen	Affects inflammatory phase by inhibiting cyclo-oxygenase production; reduces tensile strength of wound
Colchicine	Affects inflammatory phase; affects proliferative phase by decreasing fibroblast proliferation; affects remodelling phase by degrading newly formed extracellular matrix
Corticosteroids (prednisolone)	Affects haemostatic phase by decreasing platelet adhesion; affects inflammatory phase by affecting phagocytosis; affects remodelling phase by reducing fibroblasts activity and inhibiting collagen synthesis
Antiplatelets (aspirin)	Affects haemostatic phase by inhibiting platelet aggregation; inhibits inflammation mediated by arachidonic acid metabolites
Anticoagulants Heparin	Affects haemostatic phase by its effect on fibrin formation; can lead to thrombus formation by causing thrombocytopaenia (white clot syndrome)
Warfarin	Affects haemostatic phase by its effect on fibrin formation; can cause tissue necrosis and gangrene by release of atheromatous plaque emboli in form of microcholesterol crystals (blue toe syndrome)
Vasoconstrictors (nicotine, cocaine, adrenaline)	Affects proliferative phase by inhibiting neovascularisation and decreasing granulation tissue formation; impairs microcirculation and increases graft rejection and ulcer necrosis

NSAID = non-steroidal anti-inflammatory drug.

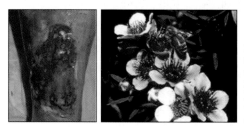

Far left: Infected leg ulcer suitable for treatment with honey. Left: Flowers from Manuka bush from which honey is extracted

Further reading

- Cullum N, Nelson EA, Fletcher AW, Sheldon TA. Compression for venous leg ulcers. *Cochrane Database Syst Rev* 2001;(2):CD000265.
- Berliner E, Ozbilgin B, Zarin DA. A systematic review of pneumatic compression for treatment of chronic venous insufficiency and venous ulcers. *J Vasc Surg* 2003;37:539-44.
- Kranke P, Bennett M, Roeckl-Wiedmann I, Debus S. Hyperbaric oxygen therapy for chronic wounds. *Cochrane Database Syst Rev* 2004;(1):CD004123.
- Eginton MT, Brown KR, Seabrook GR, Towne JB, Cambria RA. A prospective randomized evaluation of negative-pressure wound dressings for diabetic foot wounds. *Ann Vasc Surg* 2003;17:645-9.
- Karukonda SR, Flynn TC, Boh EE, McBurney EI, Russo GG, Millikan LE. The effects of drugs on wound healing—part II. Specific classes of drugs and their effect on healing wounds. *Int J Dermatol* 2000;39:321-33.

12 Recent advances and emerging treatments

Stuart Enoch, Joseph E Grey, Keith G Harding

The healing of acute wounds involves a complex and dynamic series of events leading to the repair of injured tissues. These events, triggered by tissue injury, involve four overlapping but well defined phases: haemostasis, inflammation, proliferation, and remodelling.

Haemostasis is secured by platelet aggregation and clot formation. The inflammatory phase begins with the arrival of phagocytic neutrophils and, later, macrophages at the wound site; they are important sources of and substrates for growth factors. The proliferative phase is characterised by the formation of new blood vessels (angiogenesis), synthesis of extracellular matrix components such as collagen, granulation tissue formation, and re-epithelialisation. The extracellular matrix is continually remodelled during the final phase; an avascular scar is the end result of the healing process.

Chronic wounds may be arrested in any of the four phases; commonly, however, disruption occurs in the inflammatory or the proliferative phases. Many mediators—including inflammatory cells, growth factors, proteases such as matrix metalloproteinases (MMPs), and cellular and extracellular elements—play important roles in different stages of the healing process. Alterations in one or more of these components may account for the impaired healing observed in chronic wounds.

Biological based treatments

Cryopreserved human cadaver skin (used in the UK), and human amniotic membrane and frog skin (used in other parts of the world) have long been used to treat wounds, particularly burns. More recently, artificial "skin substitutes" and growth factors have been developed to help achieve healing in chronic, non-healing wounds of varying aetiologies. These treatments target different stages of the healing process and, in the case of skin substitutes, replace lost tissue.

Artificial skin substitutes, products of tissue engineering, consist of a microengineered, biocompatible, polymer matrix in combination with cellular and/or extracellular elements such as collagen. Several growth factors (proteins involved in coordinating and regulating various interrelated processes during wound healing) produced by recombinant DNA technology have also been developed to aid healing of such wounds.

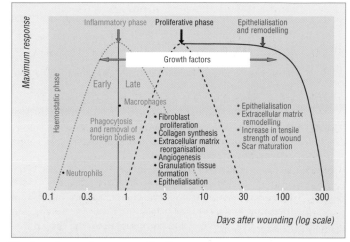

The four phases of acute wound healing

Composition of some tissue engineered skin substitutes

Product by type	Content and description
Epidermal	
Epicel, Laserskin	Cultured epidermal autograft (sheet)
CellSpray	Cultured epidermis in suspension form
BioSeed-S	Keratinocyte-fibrin-glue suspension
LyphoDerm	Lysate of cultured human keratinocytes, comprising cytokines and growth factors
Dermal (acellular)	
Integra	Two layered skin substitute comprising biodegradable matrix and bovine collagen, and outer silicone layer
AlloDerm	Processed human cadaver skin with acellular dermal matrix and intact basement membrane
Biobrane	Porcine dermal collagen bonded to semipermeable silicone membrane
Dermal (cellular)	
TransCyte	Allogenic human fibroblasts cultured on nylon mesh coated with porcine collagen
Dermagraft	Allogenic human fibroblasts cultured on bioabsorbable scaffold
Composite	
Apligraf, OrCel	Allogenic cultured skin containing keratinocytes, fibroblasts, and bovine collagen

Tissue engineered skin substitutes in wound healing

Product	Uses/advantages	Disadvantages
Epicel, Laserskin*	Permanent coverage for superficial and partial thickness burns	2-3 week lag period between biopsy and obtaining epidermis; lacks dermal component
Integra†	Immediate permanent coverage for surgically excised full thickness burns; reconstructive surgery	Requires healthy and non-infected wound base; in burns, autograft is needed after 3-4 weeks for epithelial cover
AlloDerm†	Intended to permanently cover full thickness burns and deep ulcers; reconstructive surgery	In burns, may necessitate removal after 2-3 weeks; autograft is needed for epithelial cover; not suitable for infected wounds
Biobrane†	To cover extensive partial thickness burns and donor sites	Temporary; not suitable for infected burn wounds
TransCyte‡	To cover surgically excised full thickness burns and non-excised partial thickness burns	Temporary (may need skin grafting after 2-3 weeks); not suitable for infected wounds and patients allergic to porcine collagen
Dermagraft‡	Non-healing diabetic foot ulcer and venous leg ulcer	Not for infected wounds or ulcers with sinus tracts
Apligraf§	Non-healing diabetic foot ulcer and venous leg ulcer	Not for infected wounds or patients allergic to bovine collagen
OrCel§	Acute and chronic deep dermal ulcers, partial thickness burns and donor site wounds	Not for infected wounds or patients allergic to bovine collagen

*Epidermal; †Dermal, acellular; ‡Dermal, cellular; §Composite.

Selected growth factors in wound healing*

Growth factor	Wound healing related function	Indication
VEGF	Stimulates angiogenesis and collateral blood vessel devlopment; accelerates granulation tissue formation	Has potential for use in diabetic ulcers; gene transfer encoding VEGF shown to be effective in ischaemic legs and ulcers by formation of collateral blood vessels
FGF	Promotes fibroblast proliferation, matrix deposition, wound contraction, and angiogenesis	Trials show that topical recombinant bovine FGF is effective in burns, donor site wounds, and pressure ulcers
KGF	Promotes proliferation and migration of keratinocytes	Trials show that topical recombinant human KGF-2 (repifermin) is effective in venous leg ulcers
EGF	Stimulates keratinocyte differentiation, proliferation, migration, and adhesion	Trials show that topical recombinant human EGF is effective in partial thickness burns
PDGF	Chemoattractant for neutrophils and fibroblasts; stimulates fibroblast proliferation	Topical recombinant human PDGF-BB (becaplermin) shown to be effective in diabetic foot ulcers
G-CSF	Stimulates production of neutrophils; enhances neutrophil and monocyte function; promotes keratinocyte proliferation	Recombinant human G-CSF injected subcutaneously shown to be effective in infected diabetic foot ulcers
GM-CSF	Mediates epidermal cell proliferation	Trials show that topical recombinant human GM-CSF enhances healing of venous leg ulcers
HGF	Recruits neutrophils, monocytes, and mast cells; has mitogenic and morphogenetic properties	Topical recombinant HGF may accelerate healing of chronic venous leg ulcers
TGF-β	Attracts macrophages and fibroblasts to wound site; stimulates angiogenesis and collagen metabolism	Trails show that recombinant human TGF-β2 is effective in diabetic foot ulcers

VEGF = vascular endothelial growth factor; FGF = fibroblast growth factor; KGF = keratinocyte growth factor; EGF = epidermal growth factor; PDGF = platelet derived growth factor; HGF = hepatocyte growth factor; G-CSF = granulocyte colony stimulating factor; GM-CSF = granulocyte macrophage colony stimulating factor; TGF-β = transforming growth factor β. *Only PDGF is licensed for commercial use in the United Kingdom.

Products targeting inflammatory phase

The production and activity of several proteases—including metalloproteinases, serine proteases, and neutrophil elastases, which are tightly regulated in acute wound healing—may be altered in chronic wounds. Raised levels of such proteases can be detrimental to wound healing, and products aimed at counteracting their effect have been developed. One such product is Promogran, which is designed to inactivate proteases and also protect the host's naturally produced growth factors. It may be useful in the treatment of chronic wounds refractory to conventional treatments, but it is not effective in infected wounds or those with unhealthy wound beds.

Growth factors, including granulocyte colony stimulating factor (G-CSF) and transforming growth factor-β (TGF-β), have also been used to target this phase of healing. G-CSF, an endogenous haemopoietic growth factor, induces terminal differentiation and release of neutrophils from the bone marrow, enhances neutrophil and macrophage function, and promotes keratinocyte proliferation. Recombinant human G-CSF, injected subcutaneously, has been shown to enhance healing in infected diabetic foot ulcers.

TGF-β is chemotactic for macrophages, induces the production of collagen and fibronectin, and inhibits metalloproteinase activity. TGF-β1 has been shown to accelerate wound healing in animal models, and topical application of TGF-β2 has been shown to be effective in the healing of diabetic foot ulcers

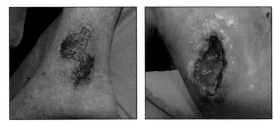

Left: Chronic venous leg ulcer suitable for protease inhibitor dressing. Right: Infected diabetic foot ulcer, associated with Charcot's arthropathy, suitable for G-CSF treatment

Products targeting proliferative phase

Growth factors

Fibroblasts, the key type of cell in the healing process, are attracted to the wound site by several growth factors, including platelet derived growth factor (PDGF) and TGF-β. They proliferate and produce the matrix proteins fibronectin, hyaluronan, and later, collagen and proteoglycans, all of which help to construct the new extracellular matrix.

PDGF attracts keratinocytes and promotes the formation of granulation tissue. Recombinant PDGF was developed to expedite the proliferative phase. Becaplermin (as Regranex gel)

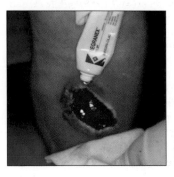

Topical application of recombinant platelet derived growth factor on a diabetic foot ulcer

is the only growth factor currently licensed for commercial use in the United Kingdom. A multicentre, double blind randomised controlled trial in patients with chronic diabetic foot ulcer showed topical PDGF to be superior to placebo in promoting healing. Its effectiveness was further enhanced when used in conjunction with debridement of the wound bed, emphasising the importance of good basic wound care.

Fibroblast growth factor (FGF) and vascular endothelial growth factor (VEGF) are active in this phase of repair. FGF promotes fibroblast proliferation and collagen accumulation and accelerates the formation of granulation tissue. VEGF plays a crucial role in angiogenesis.

Cell and matrix based treatments
Autologous fibroblasts (that is, from the patient's own dermis) seeded onto a matrix derived from hyaluronic acid have been shown to be useful in treating diabetic foot ulcers and venous leg ulcers. Similarly, acellular collagen based matrices designed to mimic the extracellular matrix have been successfully used to treat chronic ulcers of varying aetiologies.

Loss of the dermal layer occurs frequently in deep ulcers and burns. Allogenic fibroblasts, obtained from neonatal human foreskin and cultured in vitro, have been used to provide the dermal replacement in such wounds. They are seeded either on a biologically absorbable scaffold (for example, Dermagraft) or on a nylon mesh (for example, TransCyte). The proliferating fibroblasts secrete collagen, matrix proteins, and growth factors and promote healing. They are designed to provide dermal replacement in a variety of wounds, though most evidence to date comes from the treatment of diabetic foot ulcers and burns.

Processed human cadaver skin, in which the cells are removed to leave a non-antigenic dermal scaffold (for example, AlloDerm), was one of the first dermal replacement treatments. Composite skin substitutes comprising allogenic keratinocytes (epidermal equivalent) and fibroblasts (dermal equivalent) are also effective in treating diabetic foot ulcers and venous leg ulcers.

Products targeting epithelialisation and remodelling
Growth factors
Epidermal growth factor (EGF) plays a vital role in keratinocyte differentiation, proliferation, migration, and adhesion. Topical application of recombinant EGF is effective in inducing epithelialisation of partial thickness burns and superficial granulating wounds. Keratinocyte growth factor (KGF) also induces proliferation and migration of keratinocytes. Recombinant human KGF-2 induces proliferation of epithelial cells and has been shown to enhance healing of venous leg ulcers. Granulocyte macrophage colony stimulating factor (GM-CSF), secreted by keratinocytes shortly after injury, mediates epidermal cell proliferation in an autocrine manner. Topical recombinant human GM-CSF is effective in the healing of venous leg ulcers.

TGF-β3 causes reduced deposition of collagen during the proliferative and remodelling phases, thus reducing scar formation. Trials into the efficacy of TGF-β3 in the treatment of hypertrophic scars are under way; the role of TGF-β3 in the treatment of keloid scars is unclear.

Cell based treatments
Autologous keratinocyte grafts or suspension (obtained after biopsy and culture of the individual's own keratinocytes) and allogenic cultured keratinocyte grafts are used to treat diabetic foot ulcers, venous leg ulcers, and partial thickness burns. A keratinocyte suspension in a fibrin sealant matrix has recently been developed to aid adherence of the keratinocytes to the

> **Recombinant bovine FGF accelerates the formation of granulation tissue and epidermal regeneration in patients with pressure ulcers and burns. Topical VEGF improves angiogenesis and granulation tissue formation in ischaemic wounds in animal models. Intramuscular gene transfer of VEGF has been shown to improve the collateral circulation in patients with peripheral vascular disease, leading to healing of ischaemic ulcers**

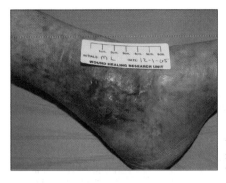

Venous leg ulcer suitable for use of dermal or composite skin substitute

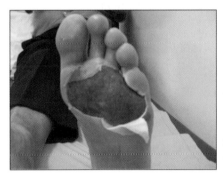

Partial thickness burn suitable for an epidermal skin substitute

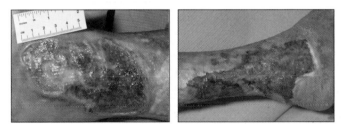

Wounds suitable for therapies aimed at the remodelling and epithelialisation phases of wound healing

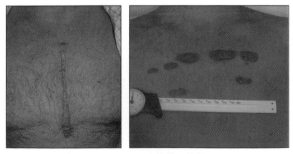

Left: Hypertrophic scar complicating healing of a sternotomy wound. Right: Keloid scarring of acne in an adolescent

wound bed (keratinocyte-fibrin-glue suspension). In addition, a total lysate of cultured human keratinocytes—comprising growth factors, cytokines, and matrix molecules, in a hydrophilic gel—has been developed to treat non-healing venous leg ulcers. The keratinocyte products are primarily used in specialist centres in the treatment of chronic wounds and burns.

Delivery of growth factors

Growth factors are currently delivered to the wound either topically (such as platelet derived growth factor) or by subcutaneous injections (such as granulocyte colony stimulating factor). However, their effectiveness is limited owing to their short half life and the presence of proteases in chronic wounds. To overcome this, gene therapy (the transfer of nucleic acid) has been investigated as a means of providing a longer lasting source

Concerns about biological products

Lack of level 1 evidence

Randomised controlled trials are lacking for many biological products, and the current evidence for many biological based treatments is based on non-randomised prospective trials, retrospective reviews, small case series (institutional or personal), and isolated case reports. Furthermore in the case of growth factors, there is little evidence on dose and duration of treatment.

No trials have evaluated the effectiveness of two comparable products (for example, dermal versus dermal skin substitute). Large, multicentre double blind randomised trials are ongoing for some of the products.

Transmission of diseases

Before human tissue is obtained for use in tissue engineered skin substitutes, the donors' medical histories are extensively reviewed and blood samples are screened for a wide variety of infectious diseases, including hepatitis, HIV, and syphilis. However, products obtained from human sources cannot be terminally sterilised owing to the presence of viable human cells, and existing tests cannot provide absolute assurance that such products will not transmit unknown diseases.

Similarly, tissue (for example, serum, collagen, cells) obtained from animal sources also carries the theoretical risk of transmitting infection, particularly prion diseases such as Creutzfeldt-Jakob disease.

Other concerns

Most biological based products contain bovine, porcine, or human constituents and thus have religious and ethical implications.

Tissue engineered skin substitutes and growth factors produced by recombinant DNA technology are expensive, which may limit their widespread use.

The wound healing chart is adapted from Clark RA. In: Goldsmith LA, ed. *Physiology, biochemistry and molecular biology of the skin.* 2nd ed. Vol 1. New York: Oxford University Press, 1991:577.

Products targeting different phases of wound healing process

Phase	Product	Growth factors
Inflammatory phase	Promogran	G-CSF, TGF-β1 and β2
Proliferative phase	Dermagraft, TransCyte, Alloderm, Apligraf, OrCel	PDGF, FGF, VEGF
Epithelialisation	Epicel, Laserskin, CellSpray, BioSeed-S, LyphoDerm, Trancell	EGF, KGF, GM-CSF
Remodelling and scarring	Silicone based products, such as silicone gel sheet (Cica-care)	TGF-β3

For abbreviations, see footnote to previous table.

Current areas of research include regulation of target genes of cells involved in wound healing; new methods of delivery of specific cell products to the wound (including nanotechnology); use of adult pluripotent stem cells, which are capable of differentiating into essential cells involved in wound healing (such as fibroblasts, endothelial cells, keratinocytes). To date, there is only experimental (though promising) evidence for gene and stem cell therapy in the treatment of chronic wounds

---

Basics of advanced wound care

- Tissue engineered skin substitutes and other biological wound manipulations are seldom effective in sloughy and exudative wounds with unhealthy wound beds
- Good wound care (wound debridement and exudate management), adequate rest, compression, pressure relief, and skin care must be provided as clinically indicated
- The new approaches and biological based treatments should complement, not replace, the tenets of good, basic wound care

---

Cutaneous wound healing is a multistep process requiring the interaction and coordination of many different cell types and molecules—including growth factors and proteases. Given the multiple molecular mechanisms involved, no single mediator, growth factor, or gene is likely to be successful in accelerating healing. Similarly, there is heterogeneity within wound types; identification of the cellular and molecular dysfunction in individual wounds and targeting or supplementing them is one of the goals for the future

---

Key references and further reading

- Singer AJ, Clark RA. Cutaneous wound healing. *N Engl J Med* 1999;341:738-46.
- Harding KG, Morris HL, Patel GK. Healing chronic wounds. *BMJ* 2002;324:160-3.
- Enoch S, Shaaban H, Dunn KW. Informed consent should be obtained from patients to use products (skin substitutes) and dressings containing biological material. *J Med Ethics* 2005;31(1):2-6.
- Jones J, Nelson E. Skin grafting for venous leg ulcers. *Cochrane Database Syst Rev* 2005;(1):CD001737.
- US National Human Genome Research Institute. www.genome.gov

Index

abrasions 17
abscess management 20, 30
acid burns 24
adhesive strips 19
Aircast boots 10
alginate dressings 26, 32–3
alkali burns 24
amputation 30
  autoamputation of toes 11
analgesics 42
angiography 11
angioplasty 7, 29–30
angiotensin converting enzyme (ACE) inhibitors 12
ankle brachial pressure index 7, 9, 11
ankle–foot orthoses 11
antibiotics 6
  infected wounds 3, 4, 36
  MRSA 38
  osteomyelitis 37–8
  side effects 37
  traumatic wounds 18
antimicrobials 41
  dressings 33
antiphospholipid syndrome 22
antiplatelets 12, 42
antiseptics 37
arterial bleeding 18
arterial bypass grafting 29–30
arterial ulceration 6–8
  allergy to dressings 34
  antimicrobial dressings 33
  iloprost 41
  management 29–30
atherosclerosis 6, 7
autoamputation of toes 11

bacteria–host interactions 36
bandages, medicated 40
barrier films 34
basal cell carcinoma 23, 30
biological-based treatments 43–6
biopsy, punch 35
biosurgery 40
bites, human/animal 18
bleach 24
blister
  burns 26
  neuroischaemic foot 10
  neuropathic foot 9
blood flow, skin necrosis 22
blood vessel intima 22
Buerger's test 7
burns 24–7
  allogenic fibroblasts 45
  artificial skin substitutes 27, 43
  assessment 25

autologous keratinocytes 45
contracture prevention 27
cooling 25
depth classification 25
major injury 26–7
management of injuries 25–7
mechanisms 24
minor injuries 26
prevention 27
referral criteria 26
superficial 25

cadexomer iodine 33
calciphylaxis 22
calcium antagonists 41
callus 3
  debridement 9
  neuroischaemic foot ulceration 10
  neuropathic foot 9
capillary bleeding 18
capillary refill time 7
casts, contact 10
cellulitis 3, 5
  foot ulceration 12
  laparotomy wound 36
  leg wound 18
cement burns 24
chemical injury 24
cleaning agents 24
clinical history taking 1
closure methods for wounds 18–19
  artificial skin substitutes 27, 43, 46
  sterile skin closure strips 17
  vacuum-assisted 10, 16, 40
coagulation factors 22–3
colchicine 42
compression bandages 6, 39–10
compression hosiery 39–40
compression stockings 6
compression therapy 6
connective tissue diseases 41
contractures
  burns 27
  scar 30
contusions 17
corticosteroids, systemic 42
cushions, pressure relieving 15

debridement 3
  arterial ulcers 30
  burn injuries 26
  callus 9
  foot ulceration 11
  honey 42
  hydrogel dressings 32
  necrotising infections 29, 36

Index

debridement (*contd.*)
  neuroischaemic foot ulceration 10
  osteomyelitis 37
  pressure ulcers 16, 29
  traumatic wounds 18
  venous ulcers 6
  see also larval therapy
dermabrasion 35
diabetic foot 1, 3, 9–12
  hydrocolloid dressings 32
  management 30
  pressure ulcers 11
  skin substitutes 45
  vacuum-assisted wound closure 10
digits
  amputation 30
  autoamputation 11
Doppler arterial waveform 9
dressings 31–4
  absorptive 34
  allergic reactions 34
  arterial ulceration 8
  burn injuries 26
  foot ulceration 10
  honey 42
  low adherent 31
  occlusive 31
  odour absorbing 4
  pressure ulcers 16
  secondary 34
  surgical wounds 19
  tightness 34
  traumatic wounds 19
  unwanted effects 33–4
  venous ulceration 6
drug therapy 41–2

eczema 3
  venous 5, 6
education, patient for foot ulceration 12
elderly patients, pressure ulcers 13, 14
electrical injury 24
electromagnetic therapy 40, 41
electrotherapy 40, 41
emollients 33–4
epidermal growth factor 45
epithelialisation phase of wound healing 45, 46
eschar 3
escharotomy 26
explosions 18
exudate 4

factitious wounds 23
factor V Leiden mutation 22
fibroblast growth factor 45
fibroblasts, allogenic/autologous 45
film dressings
  adhesive polyurethane 19
  semipermeable 31
fissures 41
flaps/flap reconstruction 20, 29
  hidradenitis suppurativa 30
  pilonidal sinus 30
  pressure ulcers 29
flash burns 24
fluid resuscitation 26
foam dressings 33
foam wedges 15
foot
  rheumatoid arthritis 21
  see also diabetic foot; neuroischaemic foot ulceration;
    neuropathic foot ulceration

footwear 10
frictional force 13–14

gangrene
  arterial ulceration 7
  dry 11
  gas 18
  wet 12
glycaemic control 12
glyceryl trinitrate 41
grafts 20
granulocyte colony stimulating factor
    (G-CSF) 44
granulocyte–macrophage colony stimulating factor
    (GM-CSF) 45
growth factors 27, 44–6
  recombinant DNA technology 46
guluronic acid 32
gunshot wounds 18

haemostasis 43
heparin 42
  necrosis 23
hidradenitis suppurativa 20, 30
honey 42
human tissue donors 46
hydrocolloid dressings 26, 31–2
hydrofluoric acid burns 24
hydrogel dressings 32
hydrotherapy 40, 41
hydroxycarbamide (hydroxyurea) 23

ibuprofen 42
iloprost 41
immobility 14
immunosuppressants 42
incisions, surgical 17
infection 3–4, 35–7
  arterial ulceration 8
  burn injuries 26
  drug treatment 41
  foot ulceration 11, 12
  microbiological analysis 35–6
  necrotising 29
  non-healing wounds 20
  pressure ulcers 16
  prevention 3
  sampling 35
  traumatic wounds 18
  treatment 36–7
  ulceration 23
  venous ulcers 6
  see also antibiotics
inflammatory disorders 21–2
inflammatory phase of wound healing 43, 46
  products targeting 44
inhalation injury 25
intermittent pneumatic compression 40
iodine 37, 41
  dressings 33
island dressings 19

keloid scars 45
keratinocyte growth factor 45
keratinocytes, allogenic/autologous 45

laboratory investigations 2
lacerations 17
larval therapy 4, 10, 16, 40
laser therapy 40, 41
leg ulcers
  compression bandages 39–40

leg ulcers (*contd.*)
  medicated bandages 40
  see also arterial ulceration; venous leg ulceration
leprosy, ulceration 42
lifting devices 15
limb amputation 30
linezolid 38
lipodermatosclerosis 5
livedoid vasculitis 41
lupus anticoagulant 22
lymphoedema 39

maggots *see* larval therapy
malignancy 23, 30, 42
malignant melanoma 33
malnutrition 15
mannuronic acid 32
Manuka honey 42
Marjolin's ulcer 23, 30
matrix metalloproteinase (MMP) 43
mattresses, pressure relieving 15
metal clips, wound closure 19
metastases 23
methacrylate superglues 19
methicillin-resistant *Staphylococcus aureus* (MRSA) 35, 38, 41
metronidazole 4, 33, 37
myiasis *see* larval therapy

necrobiosis lipoidica 21–2, 41
necrosis
  calcium antagonists 41
  heparin 23
  liquefactive 24
  warfarin 23
necrotic tissue 3
  debridement 29, 36
  foot ulceration 12
  hydrogel dressings 32
  neuroischaemic foot ulceration 10
  neuropathic foot 9
  odour 4
  pressure ulcers 16
necrotising fasciitis 29, 36
neuroischaemic foot ulceration 10–12
  metabolic control 12
  pressure ulcers 11
neuropathic foot ulceration 3, 9, 10–12
  mechanical control 10
  metabolic control 12
  pressure ulcers 11
  wet gangrene 12
nitric oxide 41
non-accidental injury 23
non-healing wounds 4
  flaps/grafts 20
non-surgical treatments 39–41
nutritional state measures 15

odour
  control 33
  necrotic tissue 4
oedema, pitting 5, 9
orthoses 30
osteomyelitis 37–8
  debridement 37
  diabetic foot 30
  diagnosis 37
  pressure ulcers 16, 29
overgranulation 4
oxygen
  hyperbaric 40
  transcutaneous 11

pain 4
  analgesics 42
  arterial ulceration 7, 8
  burns 26
pentoxifylline 41
peripheral blood flow, increase 7
peripheral vascular disease 7, 29, 41
phenytoin 42
pilonidal sinus wounds 20, 30
platelet-derived growth factor (PDGF) 44–5
pneumatic compression, intermittent 40
pneumatic devices, compression therapy 6
polyarteritis nodosa 22
polyurethane dressings 19, 33
povidone–iodine 33
pressure relieving devices 15
pressure ulcers 11, 13–16
  classification 14
  complications 16
  management 29
  MRSA osteomyelitis 38
  pathogenesis 13–14
  phenytoin 42
  risk factors 14–15
proliferative phase of wound healing 43, 46
  products targeting 44–5
protein C/protein S deficiencies 23
punch biopsy 35
purpura fulminans 23
pus sampling 35
pyoderma gangrenosum 21

quality of life, non-healing wounds 4

radiant heat dressing 40, 41
radiotherapy 23
Raynaud's disease/phenomenon 22, 41
reconstructive ladder 28–9
reconstructive surgery 28–30
remodelling phase of wound healing
    43, 45, 46
resuscitation, traumatic wounds 17–18
retinoids 42
rheumatoid arthritis 21, 41, 42

scalds 24
scarring phase of wound healing 46
scars
  contracture 30
  hypertrophic 45
scleroderma 41, 42
Scotchcast boots 10
shave therapy 6
shear force 13, 14
sickle cell ulcers 41
silicone foam dressings 33
silver compounds 37, 41
silver dressings 26, 33
silver sulfadiazine 37
skin
  artificial substitutes 27, 43, 46
  maceration 3
  necrosis 22–3
  pigmentation 5
  processed human cadaver 45
  protection 33–4
  surrounding wounds 3
skin cancers 23, 33
  malignant melanoma 33
  non-melanoma 30
skin grafting 6, 28
  see also split skin grafts

Index

slough 3
  foot ulceration 11
  hydrogel dressings 32
  pressure ulcers 16
spasticity 14
split skin grafts 26–7, 28
squamous cell carcinoma 23, 30
staphylococci 35
  see also methicillin-resistant *Staphylococcus aureus* (MRSA)
staples, wound closure 19
statins 12
sterile skin closure strips 17
streptococci 35
surgical intervention in foot ulceration 11
surgical wounds 17–20
sutures for wound closure 18–19
systemic lupus erythematosus (SLE) 22

tetanus prophylaxis 18
thermal injury 24
tissue donors 46
tissue engineering, skin substitutes 43, 46
tissue expanders, subcutaneous 28
tissue sampling 35
toe
  pressures 11
  see also digits
toenails
  arterial ulceration 7
  subungual ulceration 10
transforming growth factor β (TGF-β) 44
transforming growth factor β3 (TGF-β3) 45
trauma 17–20
tretinoin 42
triage, traumatic wounds 17–18

ulceration
  allogenic fibroblasts 45
  calcium antagonists 41
  causes 1
  iloprost therapy 41
  inflammatory disorders 21–2
  leprosy 42
  malignant 42
  mixed aetiology 8
  natural product treatment 42
  non-surgical treatment 39
  pain management 42
  pentoxifylline therapy 41
  plantar 1
  punched out 7
  risk with radiotherapy 23

types 2
  see also arterial ulceration; diabetic foot; neuroischaemic foot ulceration; neuropathic foot ulceration; pressure ulcers; venous leg ulceration
ultrasound 40, 41
  duplex 11
Unna's boot 6

vacuum-assisted wound closure 10, 16, 40
valvular incompetence 5
vascular endothelial growth factors (VEGF) 45
vasculitic ulcers 41
vasculitis
  livedoid 41
  septic 12
vasoconstrictors 42
venous haemorrhage 18
venous insufficiency 5
venous leg ulceration 5–6, 7
  autologous keratinocytes 45
  compression bandages 39–40
  foam dressings 33
  recurrence prevention 6
  skin substitutes 45
vitamin A 42

warfarin 42
  necrosis 23
Wegener's granulomatosis 22
wound(s)
  advanced care 46
  assessment 1–4
  chronic 1, 2–3, 4, 43, 45
  depth 3
  edges 2
  large open 17
  non-healing 4, 20
  reconstructive surgery 28–30
  site/size 2
  superficial swabs 35
  see also closure methods for wounds
wound bed 2–3
wound healing
  agents impairing 42
  delayed closure 28
  phases 43, 44–5, 46
  secondary intention 18, 28, 30
  systemic factors impeding 1

Z plasty 30
zinc 42
zinc paste bandages 40, 42